SELF HELP GUIDE
TO
DENTAL HYGIENE

© 2010 Leah M. Nelson

Created and written by Leah M. Nelson, RDH

Photography by Byron D. Nelson

Oral Models are Matthew Nelson and Erica Thomas

Our mouth is the doorway to the rest of the body. It delivers our words, smiles or grimaces, and feeds us. Most people tend to ignore the body in general in the absence of pain. The same is especially true for the mouth. The problem with this way of thinking is that once pain develops in the mouth the oral problem is now severe.

As a dental hygienist we have a lot of information from the experiences of helping others with their teeth. If we just had more time to share this with you these are the things we would say.

People who don't get regular dental care have a hard time understanding their mouth or what they can do at home to help themselves. By looking at the different ways problems can present in the oral cavity you can try to understand your own mouth better.

Finding the oral hygiene tools that work for your mouth and that you like to use is important. With limited patient time and multiple home care products to choose from at the store it is tough to know what or how to use them. I have provided product information to help with this.

You have every right to have questions about dental care. The dental treatment provided at the dental office by professionals for periodontal disease can sometimes be confusing to patients. At the end of this book are definitions and codes for them. That way if you want to call your dental office or insurance company about these treatment options you can talk in the dental language.

It is important to see a dentist regularly. This helps to find oral problems if they develop when they are smaller than without regular exams. When you see a professional they can diagnose and help treat dental problems. This encourages the ability for you to keep your teeth for your lifetime. The work you do at home daily is the best deterrent of gum disease and cavities. Finding the products you like and will use that work is very important. Also understanding what doesn't work, even if you use it regularly, is vital for oral health.

This book is to assist you in creating a healthier mouth. It is written in a topic format with information about each subject in the paragraph following. The information gathered is from my experience as a dental hygienist and as a dental assistant. Both the topics and explanations of them come from my 26 years of experience in the dental field. It will help you find the tools you need for better self care and be savvy on the dental treatment we provide as professionals.

TOPICS OF THE ORAL CAVITY

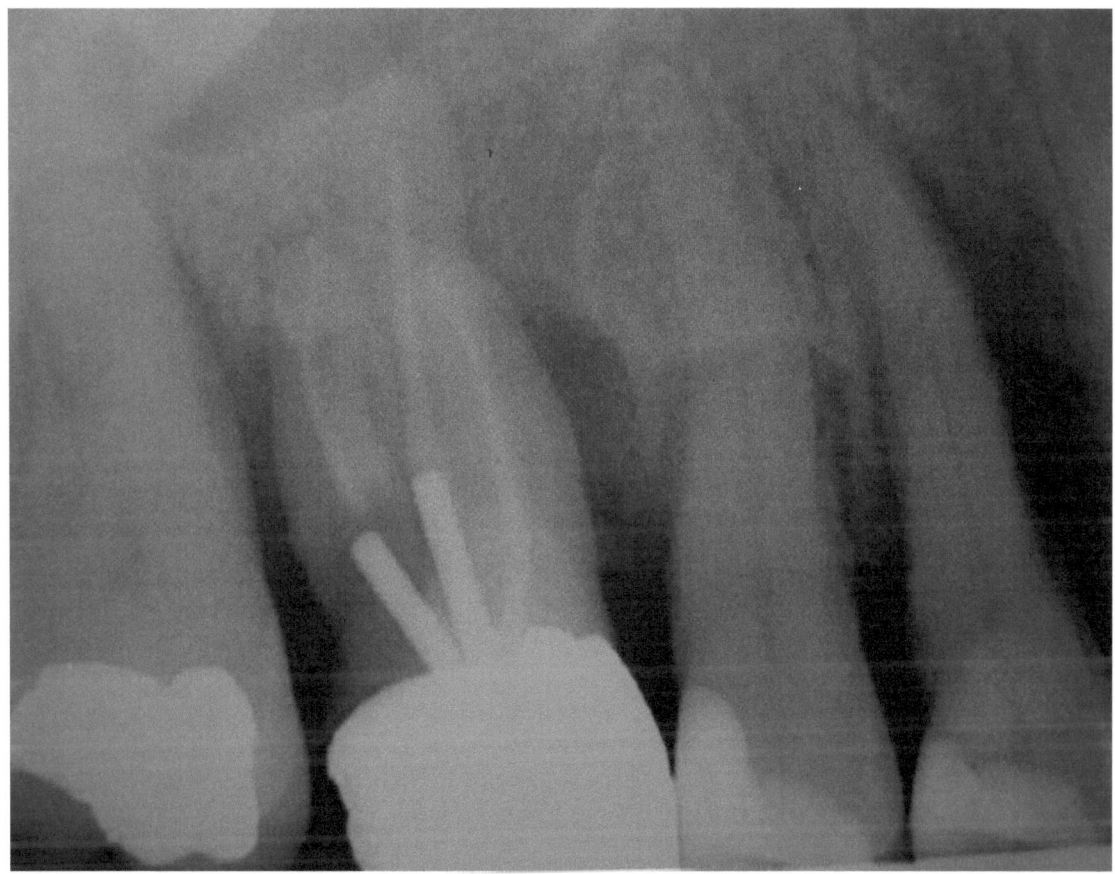

This is a digital x-ray of a person with severe periodontal disease. The bone that holds the teeth in the mouth has deteriorated down to the root tips in some areas.

Adult periodontal disease can be caused by a number of factors. Genetics, having been or currently are a smoker, immune deficiencies, lack of good oral hygiene care, lack of regularly performed professional removal of calculus, and it is communicable. The periodontal disease causing bacteria (as well as decay causing bacteria) are transmissible from person to person. Periodontal disease is the loss of bone around the teeth. This is permanent loss unless replaced by a surgeon. The bone that holds the teeth in the mouth was made in the body as it grew. These bone growing cells then died and now can not replace any loss in the mouth. This is why gum disease is so important. Keeping your teeth has shown that you will typically live longer and eat healthier than without them. We tend to be happier and more confident when we have our original teeth. While the replacement of teeth is the best it's ever been, the teeth our body grows is the best we get for chewing so we need to try to keep them. Also, the bacteria that live in our mouth that cause periodontal disease encourage other problems in the body. Research has shown they can encourage heart problems, increase the chance for acquiring diabetes, decreasing the stability of diabetes, and other health issues.

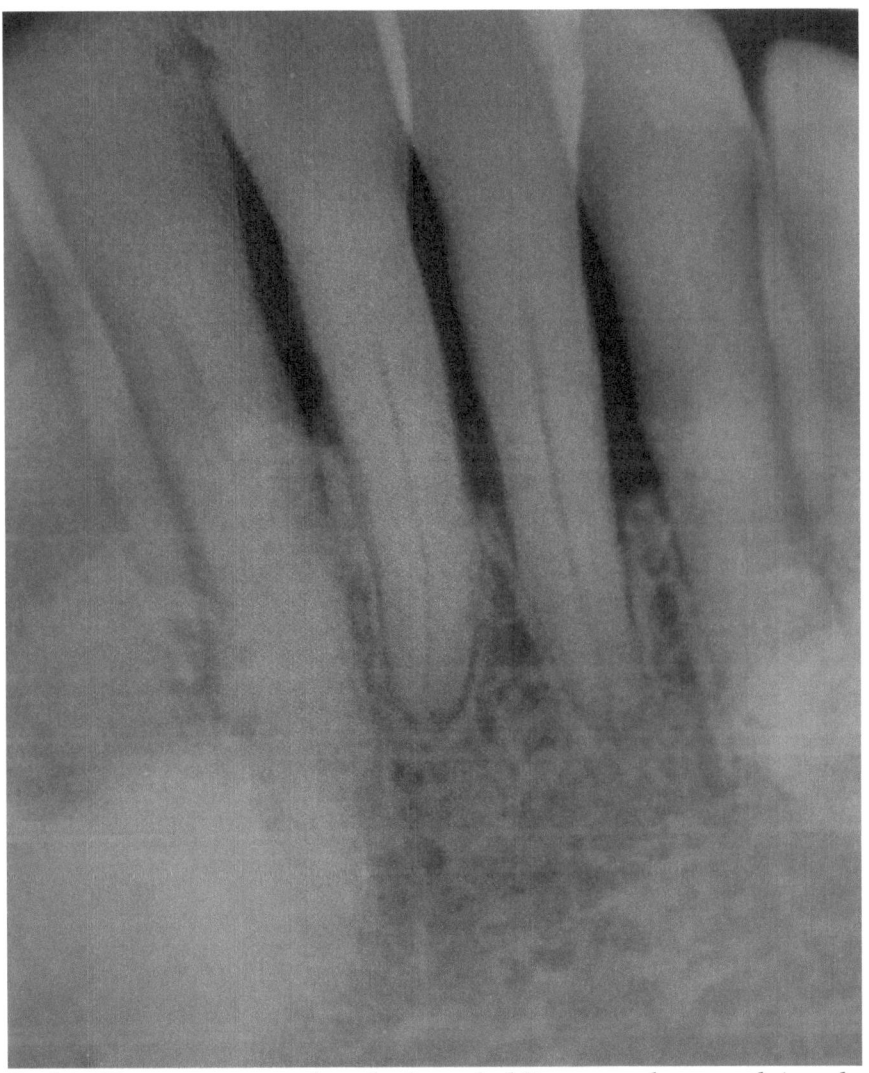

In this film you can see that the bone holding onto these teeth is only surrounding the very tips of the roots. This makes teeth loose, like a pole partially in the ground.

Mobility can be a result of permanent bone loss from periodontal disease. Because gum disease causes bone and attachment loss around the teeth, they become like trees in the ground without deep roots.

Bone loss occurs at a typical slow rate of 1mm a year, but if you have any of the inclinations toward periodontal disease this rate changes, sometimes dramatically. The length of a typical root of a tooth can be as short as 2-3mm in roots that are resorbed (something has encouraged the body to erode the root away), or as long as 14-16mm. If you loose 1mm a year then your teeth will not be there for you as an older adult.
The idea that I want you to learn from this book is that you have a lot of power to fight the infection that can develop in your mouth with periodontal disease. The different oral hygiene tools available to you will help stabilize periodontal infection. With the help of a dental professional many people can become stable and keep infection from recurring. Sometimes periodontal disease will continue to progress even with professional help or hard work at home on your teeth, all depending on the reasons for you having this disease. Take the suggestions to heart and try them, finding the ones you like that work for you, and it will go a long way to fighting the periodontal disease problem for yourself and help keep you from the transmission of it to those you love.

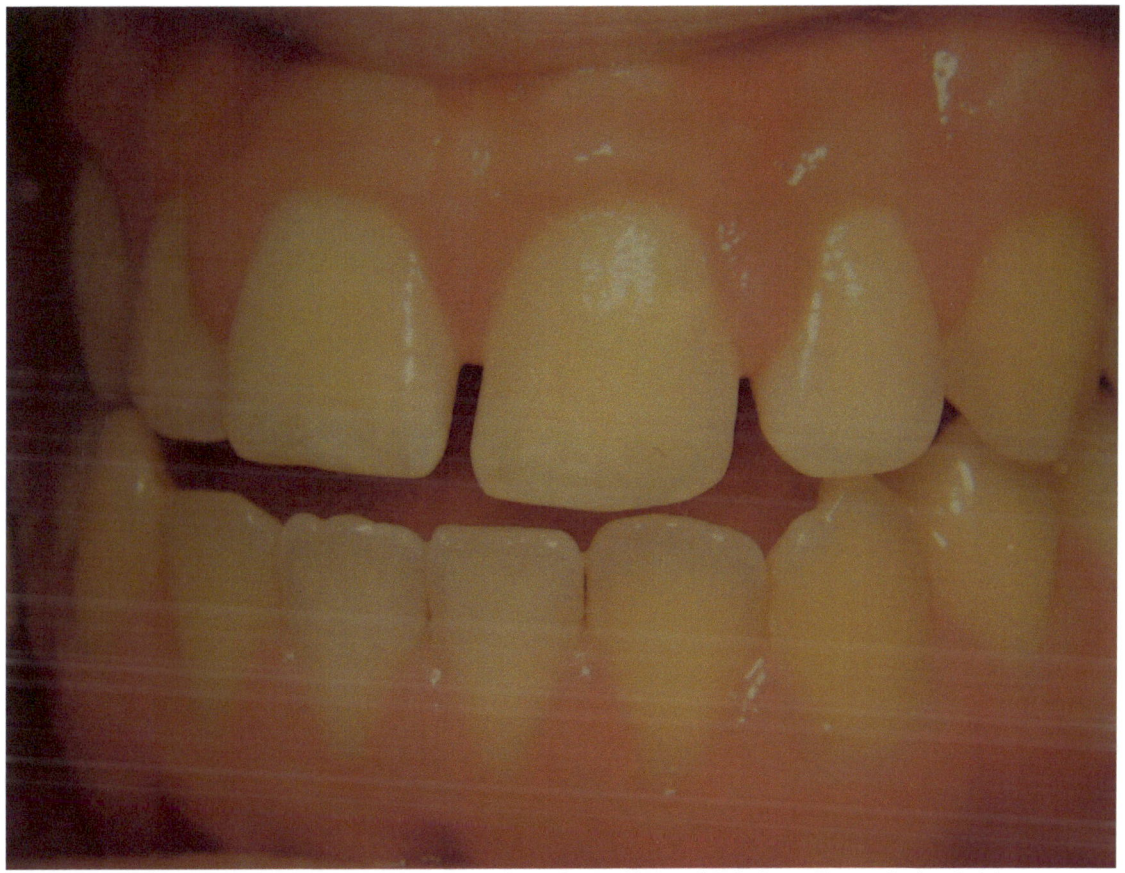

In this picture the gum tissues are round and swollen which is a sign of gingivitis.

Gingivitis is the infection of the gum tissues. When the body has an area of infection it swells with fluid, both to kill the bacteria that have accumulated there and to keep the infection from spreading. A gingival infection can come on and leave quickly due to hormones, stress, illness, and poor oral hygiene. It is treatable and can be helped much by using the tools mentioned.

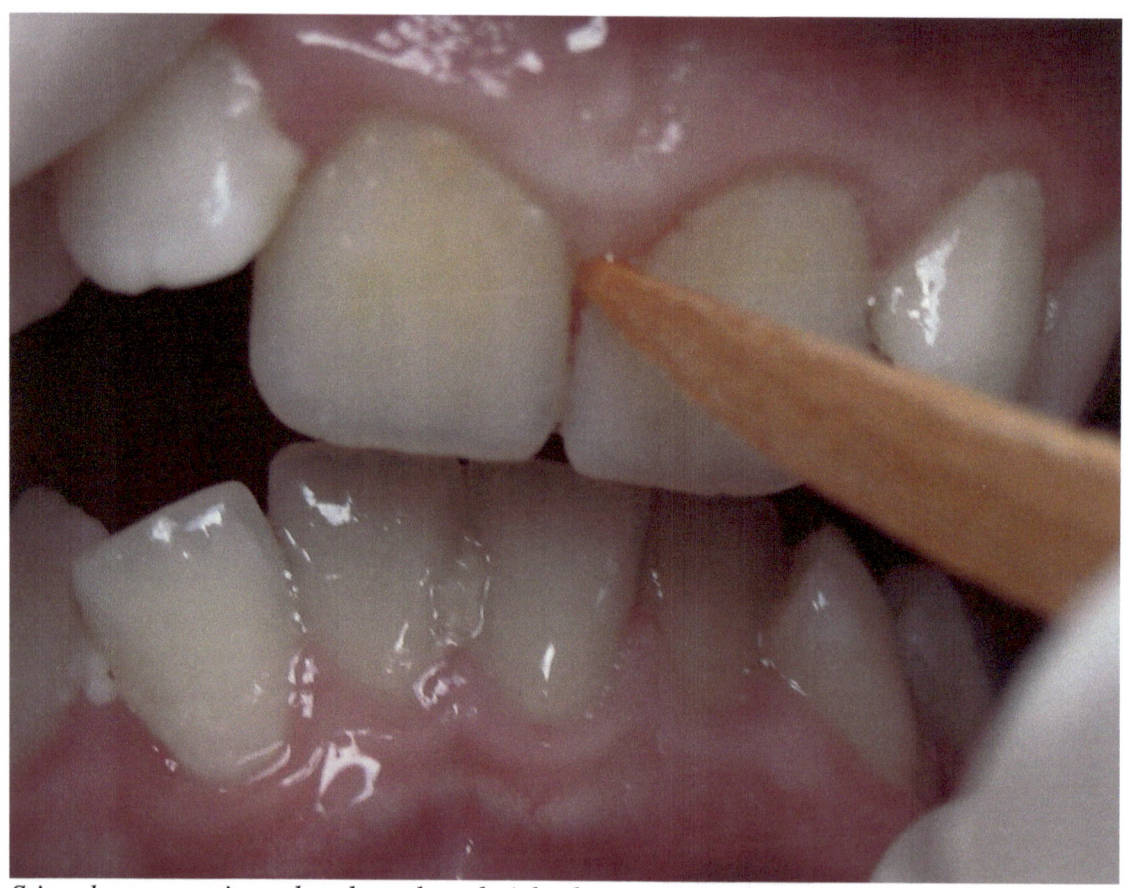

Stimudents are triangular shaped toothpicks that massage the gum tissues. When the gums are infected they can bleed with tissue massage, but this is helping them to heal.

If gum tissues are red, swollen, bleeding, round, bulky then infection is present. When the gum tissues are massaged well then blood circulates through this infected tissue. The body makes tissues swell by putting fluid there, trying to keep the infection localized. Also the fluid is trying to remove the toxic infection with specialized cells for this. By increasing blood circulation here it can remove the fluid and decrease swelling. This increases the chance for work done on your teeth at home to kill the bacteria that hide between the teeth and gums. These bacteria cause the permanent bone loss of periodontal disease. By removing the bacteria that live in our mouth regularly, you decrease the chance of the permanent loss of bone that holds the teeth in our mouth.

Juvenile periodontal disease is the loss of permanent bone that holds the teeth in the mouth on a less than adult aged person. This can occur for many reasons, as in the adult. We do see a lot of cases develop in the 13-15 year range due to hormonal changes and growth. Sometimes this can be seen by looking at the gum tissues: red, swollen, round, puffy, tall tissues. Other cases you can't tell by looking with your eyes. Juvenile periodontal disease is a challenging thing to deal with. The patient and parents need to be educated and encouraged while explaining the possible pending problems associated with lack of treatment by a professional or in changes to oral hygiene regime. Basically there is an out of control infection in their body that is causing permanent changes to their mouth. This can, more easily for a younger person than older, lead to mobility of teeth and loss of functional teeth. When the juvenile uses oral hygiene tools that work for them to massage tissues and other methods to kill the bacterial infection then the professional treatment provided will have a better chance of encouraging long term stability, hopefully halting their periodontal disease inclination.

Billions of bacteria live in our mouths. They try to hide between our teeth and gums and on our tongue because they are anaerobic which means they die with oxygen. They are constantly building homes called plaque. The sticky matrix covers and protects them. This is why disrupting the plaque all around our teeth is so important. The longer the bacteria are allowed to live in one spot, the more permanent damage they do to the teeth and surrounding tissues.

There are multiple types of bacteria that live in the mouth. Some are good and others bad. What you really want to know about them is if you disturb their homes, which is the plaque, then you expose them to oxygen which kills them. You can also kill them by using an antibacterial mouthwash. This decreases the amount of plaque/calculus being created and the amount of irritating debris that encourages gingivitis.

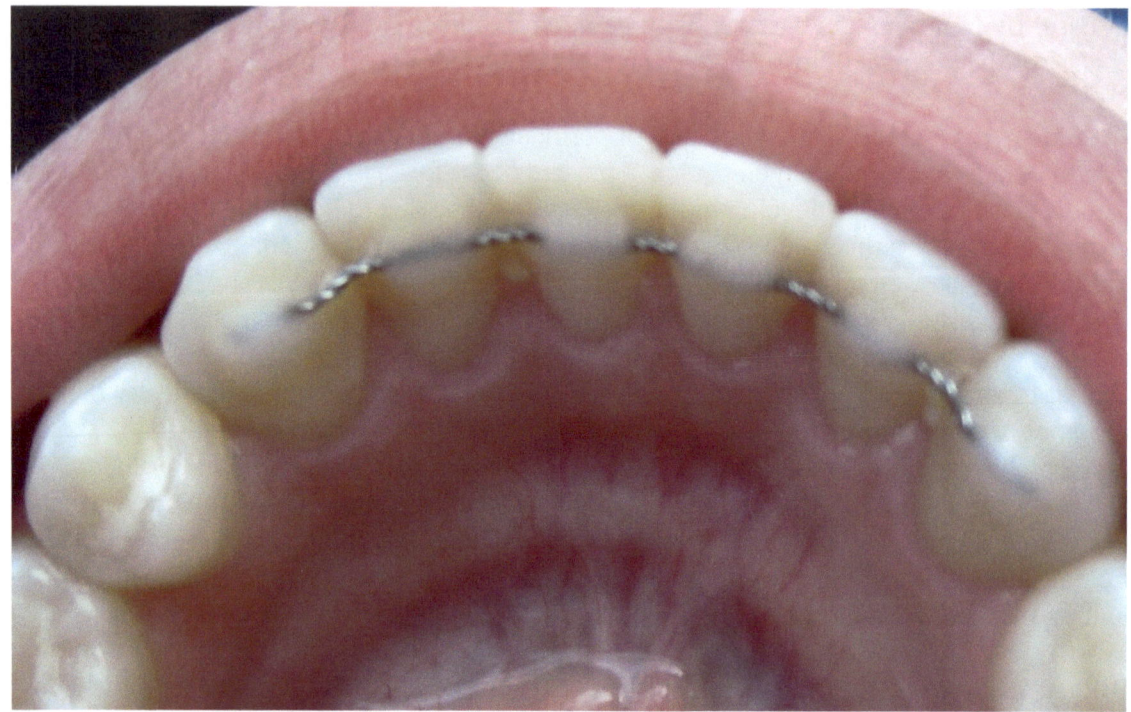

Following orthodontic treatment retainers are used to help hold teeth in place. Some are removable, this in an example of a fixed retainer. It is placed on the inside of the lower and upper front teeth. For cleaning around this area floss threaders, interproximal brushes, toothpicks, or super floss can be used.

Fixed retainers are placed following orthodontic treatment. They can be placed on inside of lower or top front teeth. There are also removable retainers to keep teeth in place.

Recession occurs when the gumline has gone below (or above for the top teeth) the enamel exposing the root of the tooth. Many things can encourage this to happen: genetics, habits of clenching/grinding/picking at the teeth, bone loss, lack or low amounts of attached tissue on the teeth, vigorous tooth brushing, or using a hard/medium toothbrush. Root exposure by itself is not usually a serious dental problem, but is a sign of problems and can encourage other negative dental issues that need to be addressed.

Recession can also encourage root decay and sensitivity to temperatures due to lack of protective covering over this part of the tooth. The roots can be covered with tooth colored fillings if needed. They can be covered with a varnish of fluoride at your dental office that can help with sensitivity, although usually temporarily due to this wears off. MI paste and desensitizing toothpastes can help with sensitivity to temperatures. Night guards can protect the tops of teeth if you grind your teeth and sometimes can stop grinding. If you have a lack or low amount of attached tissue on a tooth a surgeon can replace this tissue either from your own mouth or artificially. A hard or medium toothbrush is like using a wire brush on your teeth. Teeth are curved and these bristles do not bend or flow between the teeth well. The harder bristles only scrub the tip of the teeth that they are brushing, helping to permanently remove tooth structure.

Smoking encourages periodontal disease by decreasing the health of the good bacteria in our body. It also dries the mouth encouraging the bacteria's' ability to stay in one place, creating more plaque and calculus. This also is what stains stick to, making the teeth discolored.

Diabetes decreases our ability to fight infection in the body. Periodontal disease and gingivitis are oral health problems that can be easier to acquire and harder to control with diabetes.

Long in the tooth is the process of periodontal disease encouraging bone loss then the gum tissues following this bone line encouraging more tooth exposure and the tooth looking long as a result.

Interproximal Papilla is the area between the teeth that comes up toward the contact of the teeth. If there is no contact or an open space between the teeth then papilla are inclined to continue to stay swollen without regular tissue massage. By increasing blood circulation to interproximal tissues it takes away fluid and swelling helping you to reach the bacteria that live between the teeth and gums. These hiding bacteria are the ones that cause gum disease and are anaerobic=die with oxygen.

Flossing only cleans 2-3mm into pockets between teeth and gums. If you have periodontal disease you have pocket depths that are deeper than this and why simply flossing will not kill all bacteria that live in the deepest pockets. The addition of other tools can supplement your homecare regimen for helping to stabilize periodontal disease.

Yeast in mouth occurs when the balance of good-vs-bad bacteria in the mouth gets off. This can happen from bactericidal mouthwash or a decrease in immune system from stress or disease. Candidiasis is treated with an oral rinse or lozenges. You also want to stop using mouthwash until the yeast is gone, sometimes indefinitely. Yeast infection in the mouth can look many different ways. It can be a black, hairy tongue; whitish coating on tongue; very red tissues; and can be sore to no sensitivity from it at all. Sometimes yeast can cause a bad taste in the mouth or it will feel coated.

Dry brushing means using a toothbrush prior to placing water or toothpaste on it to brush the teeth. It makes the bristles more stiff and able to scrub stain and plaque off better. Then you should place toothpaste on your brush and brush all your teeth. This can be a good way to massage the tissues between regular brushing.

Carrying oral hygiene devices with you encourages their use. The human condition is out of sight, out of mind. If you see it, find it, come across it, you will use it. Strategically placed oral hygiene tools will get used. Place these tools in areas you will be regularly. Some examples are near a computer, television, nightstand, shower, toilet, car, in purse or wallet and they will be used.

Hormonal gingivitis can occur whenever there is a change in hormones. Hormones feed the bacteria that live in our mouth. The decrease in hormones decreases the strength of our good bacteria that fight infection. This helps gingivitis causing bacteria to flourish. As women we have many opportunities to develop this. Examples of this are puberty, taking birth control pills, our "time of the month", pregnancy, nursing, and menopause. Men have their times, too. These are mostly during their fast growth times of life.

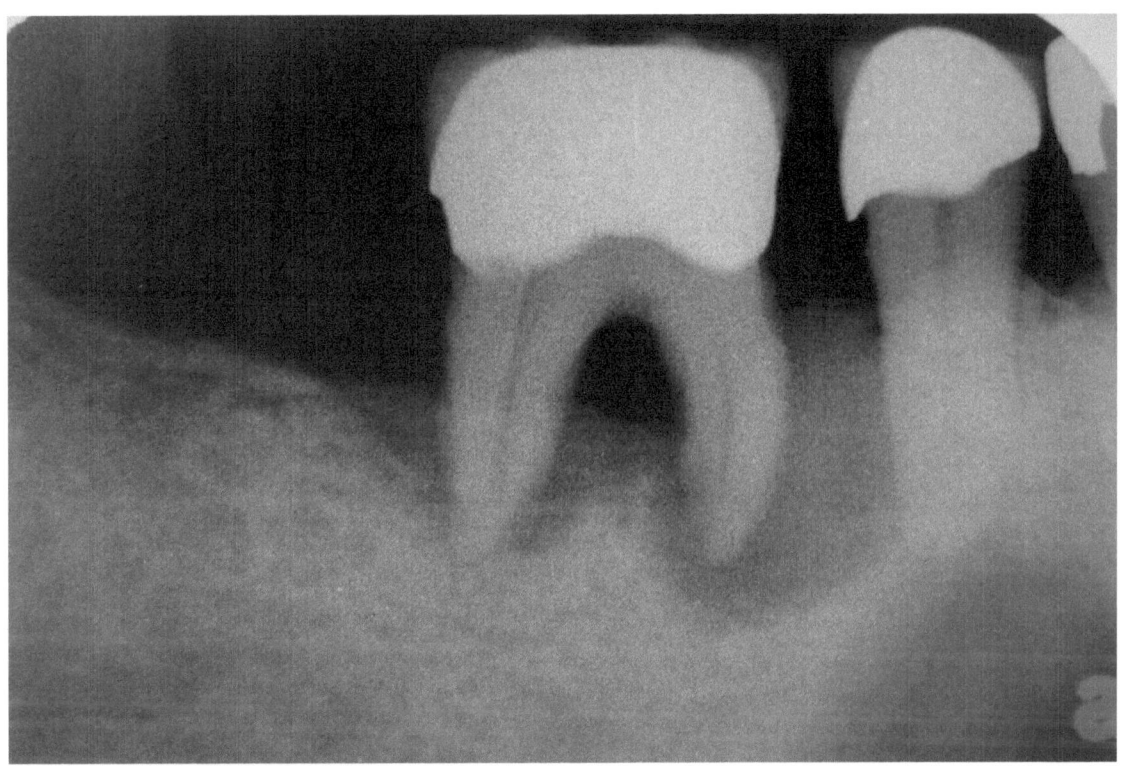

Periodontal abscess is infection in tissues from periodontal disease causing bacteria. This can be treated by a dental professional by thoroughly removing debris, bacteria, and roughness in the area as well as with antibiotics orally taken or placed by powder in a tube under the tissues.

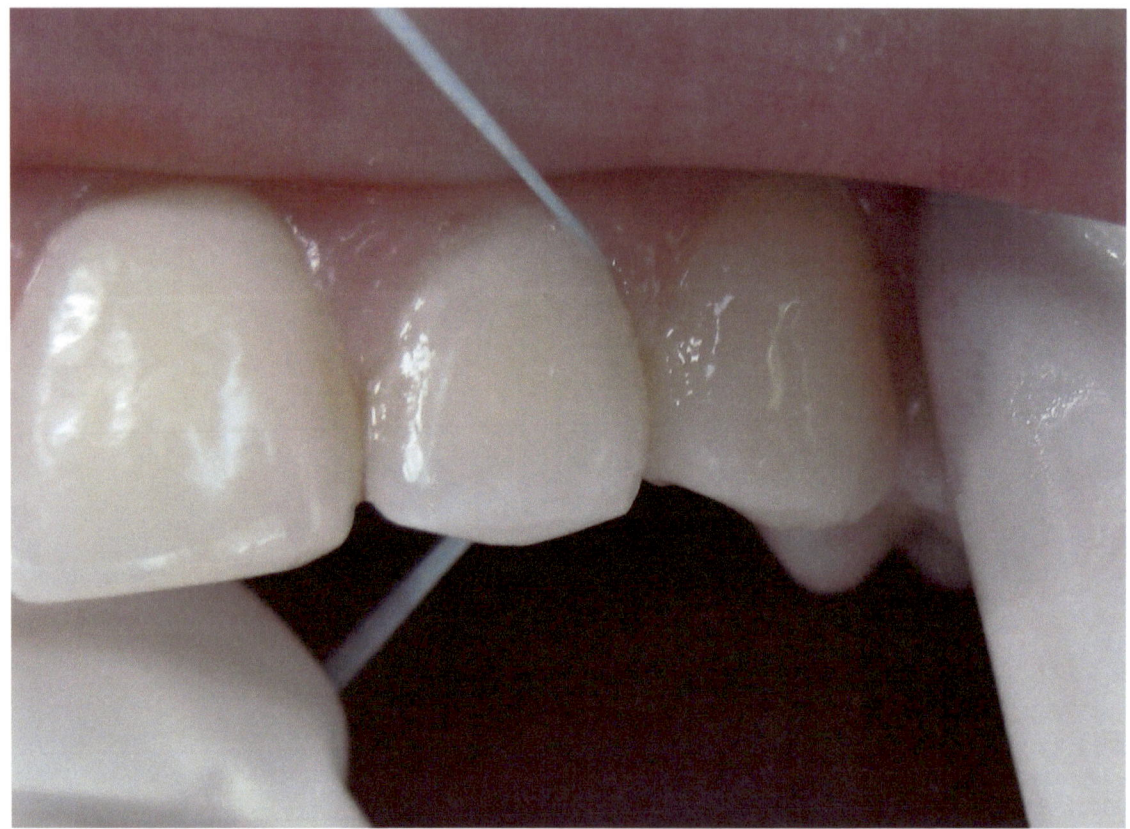

Without proper use under the gumline floss does nothing to fight gingivitis or periodontal disease.

Floss cuts happen when we don't curve well around our teeth when flossing. They usually heal but sometimes are so deep they don't. You are better just to take your time and curve to scrub under the gum tissues.

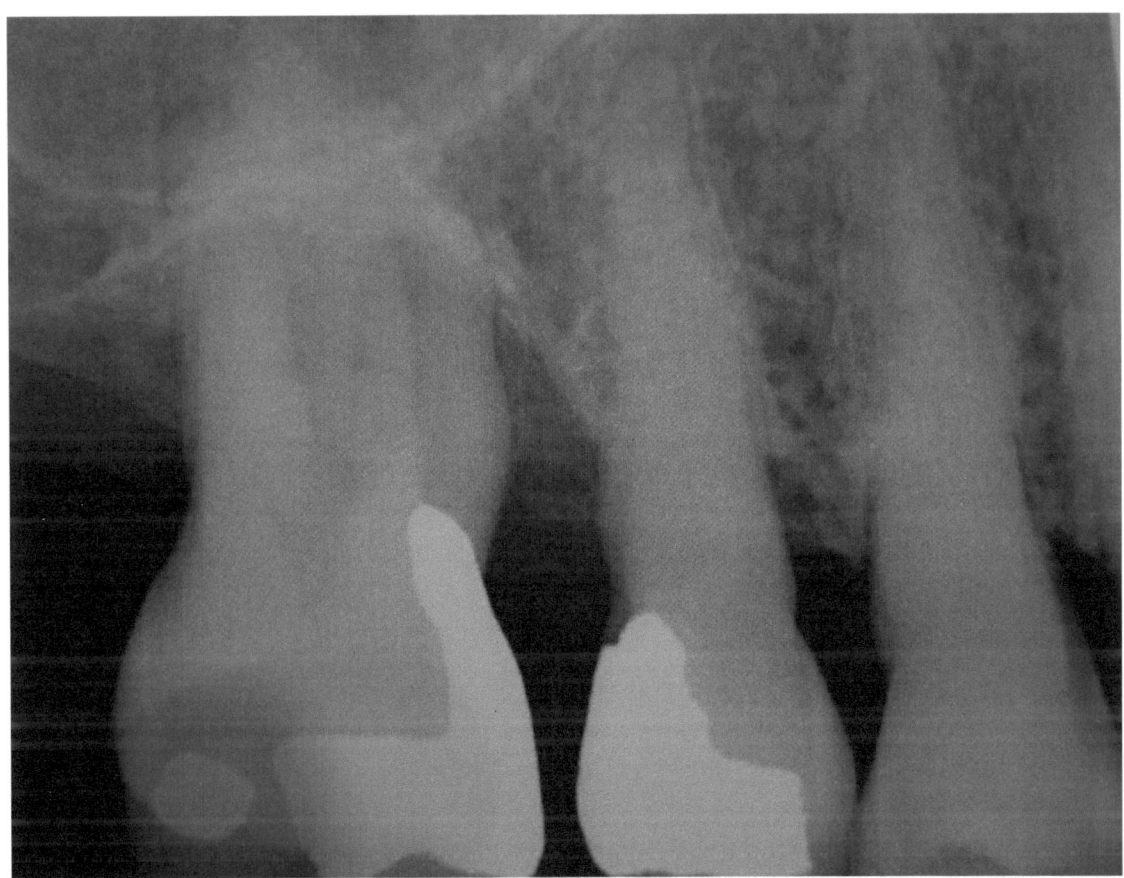

The bone levels on these teeth are below where it should be. This is caused from periodontal disease.

Dental professionals are here to help. We can measure your gum tissues for periodontal disease, notifying you of how you stand and the problem areas of your mouth. We can customize your home care regimen for just what you need to help you with your personal oral health issues. The removal of calculus and smoothing of roots is the treatment provided to decrease the ability for bacteria to colonize and continue to create infection in the mouth.

Pocket depths are the only way to measure and check regularly the amount of bone loss and tissue swelling a person has at that moment. With multiple measurements by the same provider over time progression or healing can be noted and observed precisely. As dental professionals we use a small ruler to measure from the top of the gum tissues to the bottom of the pocket between the gums and tooth. Your measurements can be explained to you, helping each person to know their status. This is priceless for helping each person to take care of their problem areas with the best tools for them. This is why flossing is not the only oral hygiene tool available for caring for your teeth. Each homecare product has its uses. Every person has things they will use and tools they won't. We have to work with each patient as an individual based on their eagerness to try products and disinterest in using others.

Frequent recalls are recommended for frequent removal of bacteria in the deepest pocket depths before further destruction to the bone can occur. The length of time for the bacteria to begin causing permanent destruction in deeper pocket depths is about 90 days.

Gums bleed due to sores that have developed on the inside pocket lining between the teeth and the gums. This occurs due to irritants that are toxic to the tissues (bacteria, plaque, and calculus). When your gums are infected scabs develop on the inside of the tissues which come off when fluid tries to escape from these infected tissues. If your gums bleed they are not healthy. Tissue massage is an important part of healing these tissues and help rid gingival of infection, just like it would in any other part of our body.

Exudate is another word for pus. It develops in tissues that are infected. It is green or yellowish in color and comes out between the teeth and gingiva. This chronic infection is very unhealthy. The pus can be released sometimes just from massage with your finger. It is important to see a dental professional if you notice this. There are many things a professional can do to help with this disease process.

Plaque are the homes of the bacteria that live in our mouth. You know that furry feeling on your teeth in the morning? These are the condominiums of your oral bacteria, trying to live on your teeth. If you don't disturb their homes they continue to create plaque, acid, and become worst types of bacteria. The plaque left undisturbed for on average of 24 hours begins to crystallize. It forms crystal structures from the calcium and phosphorous in our saliva. There are saliva glands right behind the lower front teeth and outside of upper back teeth that encourages buildup here, especially. The inside of the lower front teeth is every mammals worst calculus building area due to anatomy and difficulty in being able to clean here. The ability of plaque to calcify is dependent on the level of acidity in the mouth. This is generally genetic, although can be changed by the intake of acidity in the oral cavity. Commonly a person is either acidic and gets cavities easily or more basic and their plaque hardens more quickly into calculus or tartar.

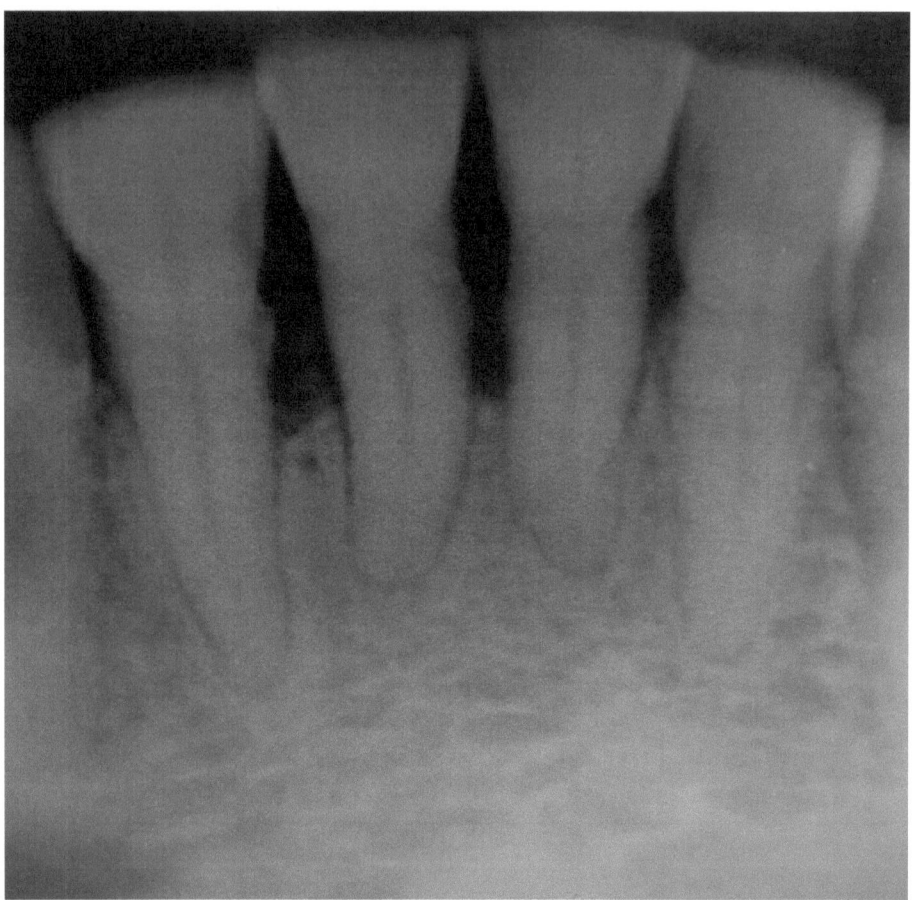

The bumps on the sides of the teeth here is calculus on the roots.

Calculus forms above and below the gum tissue line. Everyone grows some calculus on their teeth. It is a structure attached to the tooth that the bacteria live on. It is not easily destroyed so the bacteria are able to live longer undisturbed here, causing bone and tissue destruction easily. Once calculus bonds with the tooth it can be removed only by a dental professional by multiple means.

Most stain on the outside of teeth develops by either poor oral hygiene or introducing to the mouth a staining food or liquid. Some ways to fight extrinsic stain are with dry brushing, using whitening toothpastes or mouthwashes, bleaching treatments, or using an abrasive dentifrice like baking soda.

Straws are great for getting staining, acidic, sugary liquids past the teeth decreasing these affects on the oral cavity. Liquids encourage decay by feeding the bacteria that cause oral problems. Every time we take a sip the bacteria living in our mouth eat and create acid for 20 minutes.

Orange and green stain occurs when a person doesn't clean their teeth sufficiently to remove all plaque and bacteria. These stains are mold-yes, mold does grow on teeth.

Some stains are from ingesting high amounts of fluoride when teeth were being made by the body creating a mottling affect. This can be white or dark on the tooth and is permanent. It can be covered with composite or porcelain veneers or crowns. Other stains are from ingesting forms of tetracycline when teeth are being created. These are also permanent. Sometimes bleaching can help this, sometimes not. It is best to see a dental professional for advice about this. These teeth can also be covered by veneers or crowns.

Getting older is better than not, but can encourage oral health issues. Xerostomia/dry mouth, periodontal disease, root decay are the most common dental concerns as we age.

Medications can change the oral condition. Many medicines, especially the most commonly used ones, encourage dry mouth. Some medications encourage tissue growth. Others help plaque to calcify more quickly. Recently a well known medication for osteoperosis has been shown to encourage jaw bone cell neucrosis where the cells die in the bone. We should always be aware of the possible side effects of the medications we are taking.

Xerostomia means dry mouth. Many people suffer from this and I mean suffer. This problem changes your ability to taste, kiss, and encourages teeth discoloration. It also helps to progress decay, sometimes very quickly. The dryness keeps the oral bacteria from being moved around so their acidic environment stays in one place for a longer period of time. This problem is caused by age, many different medications, mouth breathing/allergies/snoring. In general products for this either cover the teeth, strengthen the outside of the teeth, or try to encourage saliva flow without feeding the bacteria that live in the mouth. There is artificial saliva that is more viscous than biologically created saliva therefore coating the teeth. You place a couple of drops under your tongue and rub it around on your teeth. This helps protect the teeth from decay causing bacteria. Fluoride prescription toothpastes or mouthwash can be recommended to strengthen the outside of the teeth. This makes it more difficult for the acidic bacteria to create cavities. Other products for dry mouth include lozenges and gum with xylitol. This is an artificial sweetener that oral bacteria can not eat. It also retards their ability to consume other sugar, helping to kill them.

Mouth breathing and snoring dries the mouth due to air flowing over the teeth. This is especially true for the top and lower front teeth. When dry the teeth are sticky and can acquire plaque, stain, and calculus more easily. Because plaque and calculus are homes for the bacteria to live on our teeth, and they are constantly creating an acidic environment, it is an irritant and encourages swollen, bleeding gum tissues. Therefore mouth breathers should especially brush their front teeth and gum tissues well.

Bacterial endocarditis or infection in the blood stream can occur due to poor OH/HC from bacteria or dental procedures. People with certain health issues need an antibiotic pre-medication prior to dental treatment. This is because the type of bacteria that causes endocarditis only live in the mouth and are introduced to the blood stream easily. You should consult the American Heart Association to be sure of current guidelines.

Youth caries with it sometimes a feeling of invincibility but gum disease can affect us at any age. Lack of good oral hygiene, defiance of authority that educates, growth and puberty hormones, as well as higher occurrence of orthodontic treatment make it easier to develop gingivitis, periodontal disease, and decay. Regular professional care encourages self care and awareness.

Sonic toothbrushes use vibration to clean the teeth. This motor movement breaks away plaque better than our manual brushing. The sonic toothbrush has also been shown to be less destructive to exposed root surfaces than our muscles and a toothbrush. By providing a better gum tissue massage the electric tooth brush also helps decrease tissue swelling. With disabilities or age our grip and dexterity with a manual decreases so an electric toothbrush is ideal for removing plaque and bacteria growth.

Manual toothbrushes are good at having more control over brushing. This can be good for anatomical concavities or convexities (curves in or out). Some people do not like the motorized movement of an electric toothbrush

Wisdom teeth can cause permanent bone loss around the teeth in front of them if they are impacted. Even if they are sideways wisdom teeth still try to come into the oral cavity so if they are facing towards the teeth in front of them it can cause the bone on the back of those teeth to go away.

Braces decrease the ease of removing bacteria and plaque from the teeth which can encourage decalcification and gum disease problems. Decalcifications are the permanent scars from the acidity of bacteria and plaque on the teeth. It is basically a cavity that you can see. It looks white at first but with progression turns black and can chip the enamel off in that area.

Grinding can encourage breakdown of the bone that hold the teeth in the mouth. This can make the gum tissue line go below the root line exposing this area of the tooth. It also wears the top of the teeth, changing aesthetics of the smile as well as the longevitiy of the teeth in the mouth.

Trauma to the face/teeth encourages multiple dental problems. Many times a root begins to die with the trauma but signs do not develop for years. Some signs of this are a singular discolored tooth, abscess/infection at base of tooth, or a loose tooth.

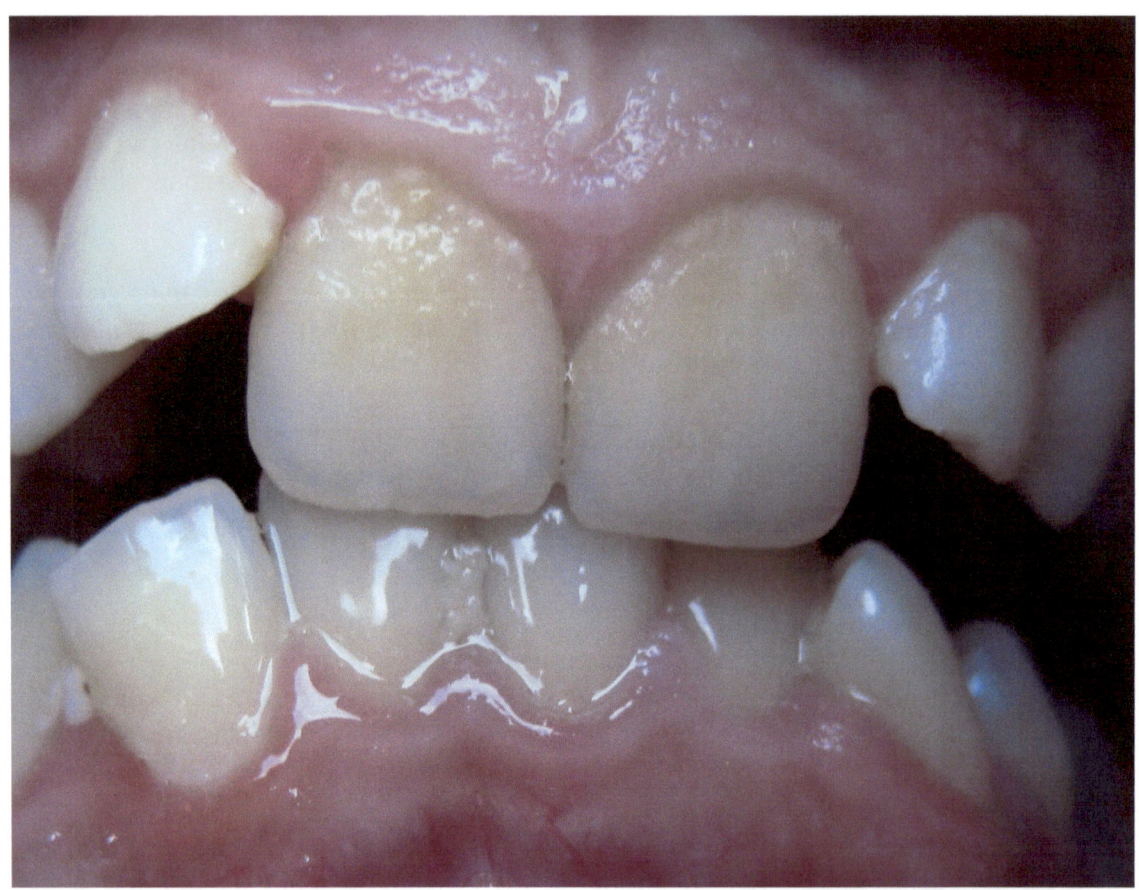

Plaque tends to accumulate where teeth touch. You can see the yellow plaque at the gumline as well. Millions of live bacteria live there and are happily being acidic and destructive.

Bacterial colonization occurs when bacteria is left undisturbed for 24 hours.
It is important to clean our teeth after we eat. Food not only feeds our body but also the bacteria in our mouth. Due to the mouth being the first place digestion begins it is a very acidic environment. If we can remove the food and plaque created by the bacteria living in our mouth then cavities are harder to have occur.

Alcoholism increases the acidity of the oral cavity so that decay occurs more easily. The enamel gets eaten away by the alcohol and an alcoholic's poor health decreases the strength of the helpful bacteria in our mouth, allowing periodontal disease causing bacteria to flourish.

Drug use is also acidic and encourages holes/cavities to develop in the teeth.

Overhangs are bulky fillings or crowns at the point of intersection with the tooth. If the dental work has extra material under the tissue it traps bacteria just like calculus. This will irritate the gum tissues and can encourage decay and permanent bone loss.

Crowns are wonderful at holding a tooth together. This treatment is recommended when a tooth can not be filled successfully with material but must be overlaid with a lab created fixed material. Crowns are made of porcelain, porcelain with metal underneath, or gold. When they fit right it can look and feel like the original tooth.

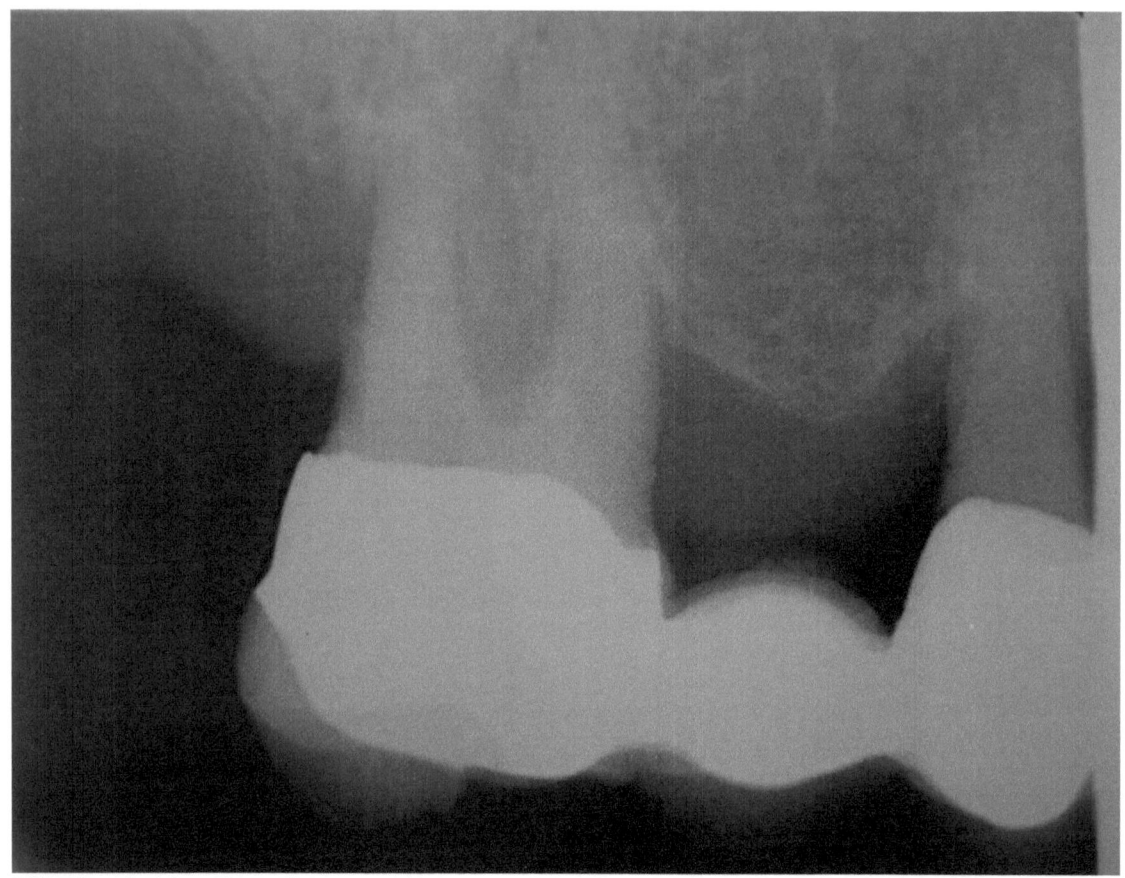

This is a bridge. It replaces a missing tooth in the center. The ends of the bridge are crowns.

Tooth removal is always the last resort from a dental professional's perspective. Keeping your teeth increases the quality and length of life according to research. We want to help encourage and educate people so that this becomes an important part of keeping themselves healthy.

When a tooth is lost there are multiple ways to close the space. One is to have a bridge placed. Depending on the space that is to be filled it can be a connecting bridge from one tooth to another if a tooth is lost between them. Crowns are placed on the teeth opposite the missing tooth with a solid bridge area in the middle that looks like a tooth. There is a slight space under here that needs to be cleaned regularly. If it is not then decay and bone loss can be encouraged. The bridge is fixed and not removable.

Another way to replace a lost tooth is with implants. These replace the lost tooth with a titanium screw that is placed in the jaw bone, where the roots of the lost tooth used to be. Then a crown is made to go over the implant. The success rate on implants is 90% and continues to increase.

Partials or flippers replace teeth with a removable device. These tend to be less expensive than the other options but can lead to other problems. They are acrylic and fit around teeth so can encourage plaque to build on the teeth that the partial sits against. They need to be removed and cleaned well at night so the tissue under these appliances can breathe and not have the irritating plaque rubbing against it all the time.

Dentures are placed when an entire arch of teeth must be removed. These are typically more comfortable for the top teeth than the bottom due to having suction to keep the denture from moving from the roof of the mouth. They do have implants that can be placed to fit an overlaying denture onto. This increases the fixation of the appliances increasing their comfort and chewing ability. Having implants in the bone also helps to keep the mandible or lower jaw from becoming thin from lack of blood circulation after tooth loss.

Carbohydrates turn into sugar which feeds bacteria so carbohydrates that stick; such as potato chips, crackers, bread; are especially decay encouraging. It is best to remove this food as soon as possible after consumption.

Sugar feeds bacteria so they create acid for 20 minutes after every bite or sip. If food is left on teeth then the acid creation continues until 20 minutes after food is removed. Try to brush, floss, rinse or use a straw to decrease this decay causing problem.

Pop causes three oral problems: acidity, stains on teeth, and/or decay from sugar. All these can be decreased by using a straw with any liquid that encourages these issues. Sugar pop has multiple tablespoons of sugar per can, up to 12 tablespoons in some. Energy drinks encourages the same problems as soda pop.

Rinsing at bedtime is the best way to decrease oral health problems that love the lack of saliva flow during sleep and snoring.

Cancer in or around mouth can look very different. If you chew tobacco or smoke you want to make sure your dentist is providing regular oral cancer screenings to look for tissue changes or abnormality

As dental professionals we really do want you to be comfortable during dental treatment. It you are relaxed we can provide better dental work for you. This comfort during dental treatment can be provided in many ways. Nitrous is a gas you breathe in the office. It works to relax you while you breathe it. The oxygen is always above the amount in the air around us so it is safe to use. There is also a long lasting topical gel, a couple of different numbing rinses, and a gel that can be placed between the teeth and the gums for anesthetic. Headphones with music and even televisions can be found in dental offices for distraction.

ORAL HEALTH AIDS

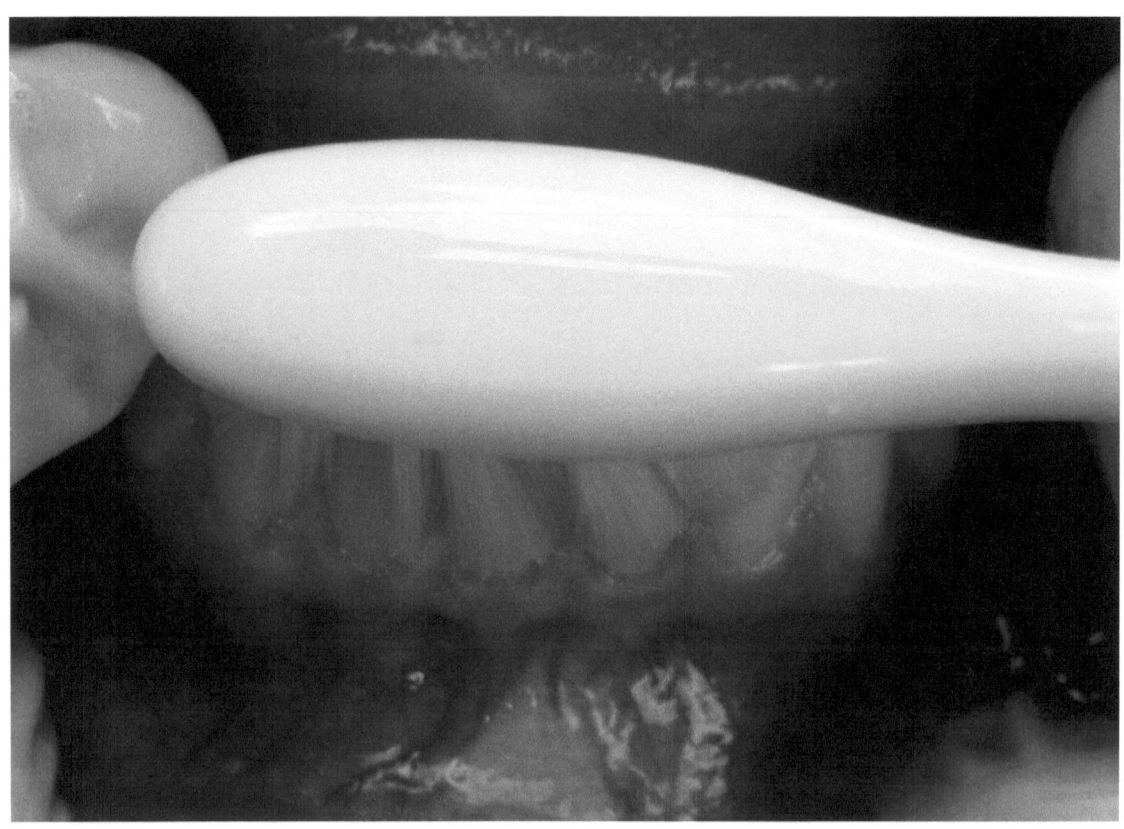

Bass brush method is the preferred method for brushing your teeth and gums. By angling your toothbrush, manual or electric, toward the gums you will massage them. Keeping gum tissues massaged helps decrease fluid that develops there as well as lessens plaque and bacterial irritants to the tissues that encourage swelling.

Manual toothbrushes come in different bristle strength as well as shape at end of bristles. The shape of bristle groups, tip at end of brush, items added to sides of brush, and other additions change a toothbrush. Patients can be confused about which toothbrush to get or what is best. The basics are softer bristles cause less destruction to the teeth and gums around them. The rounded bristle tips are gentle so preferred. Smaller toothbrushes tend to clean back teeth better. Other additions can be judged per patient.
Positives=less expensive than a motorized brush.
Negatives=can be more destructive to teeth and tissues around them than the electric toothbrushes.

Sonic toothbrushes are made by multiple brands. The differences between them tend to be toothbrush size and addition of vibration speed or length of time. You can purchase rechargeable sonic toothbrushes which are more expensive than the replacement battery operated sonic brushes. They use vibration to break off the debris on the teeth which helps us to have less plaque on our teeth. The vibration massages the tissues and can help with gingival swelling.
Positives=removes plaque more quickly than manual brushing.
Negatives=not as portable as a manual toothbrush, and more expensive than a manual or spin brush.

Spin brushes cost a little more than a manual toothbrush, less than a sonic one. The motorized movement of bristles helps to remove plaque better than manual toothbrushes.
Positives=movement of bristles help remove plaque better than a manual toothbrush.
Negatives=tend to have a large toothbrush head which can make it more difficult to reach back teeth well.

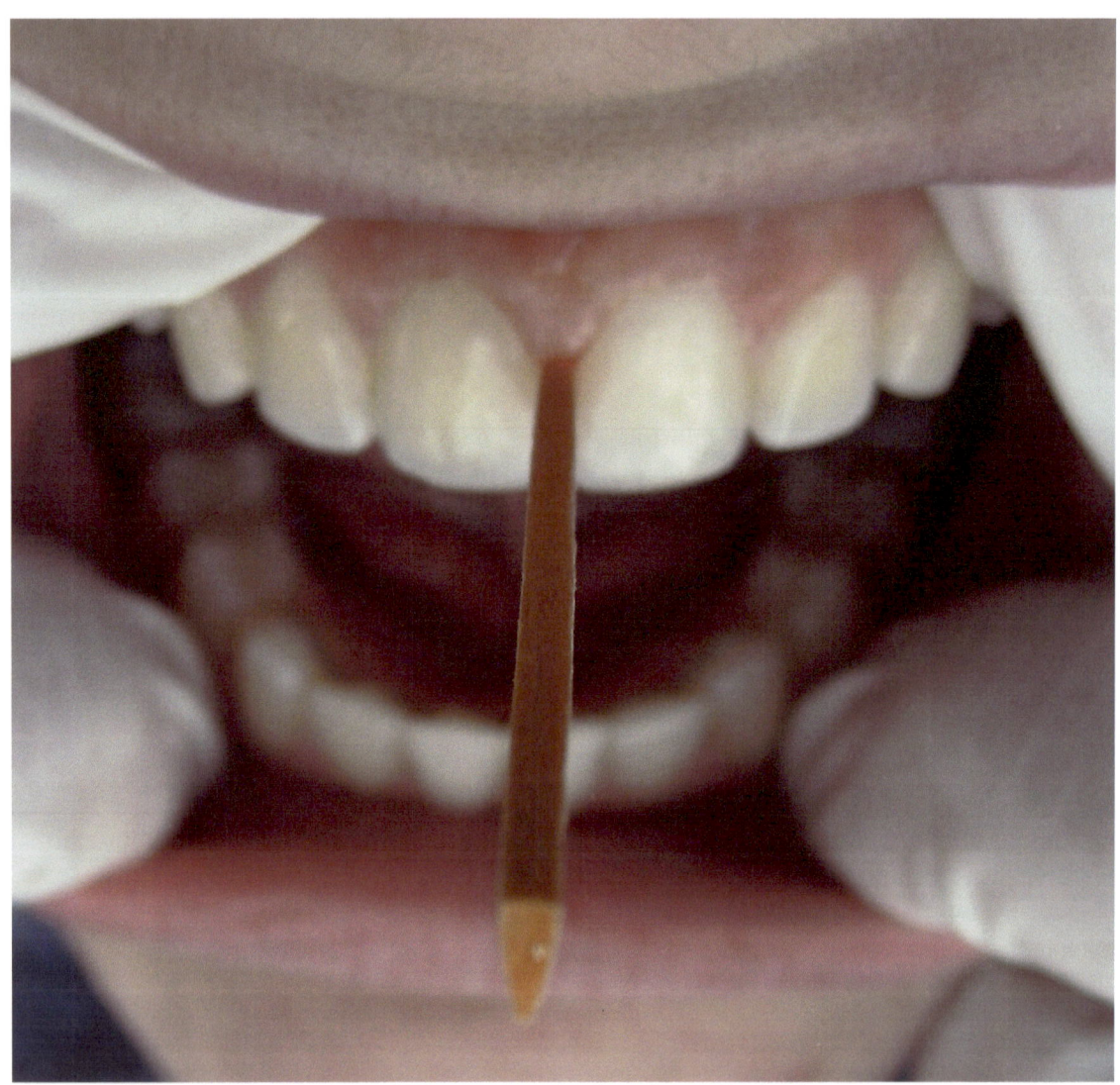

Because Stimudents are shaped like a triangle they fit easily in the space between the teeth. The flat side of the triangle is the end that goes against the tissues. When using them on the top teeth, the flat side goes up. For the bottom teeth the flat side goes down.

Stimudents are toothpicks shaped like a triangle that come in a matchbox size case. They break off individually and are used to massage the gum tissues. In use you have to place the flat side of the triangle against the tissue so take a little conception of this for proper manipulation. Made of birch wood they are softer than round toothpicks and have a little give to them.

Positives=Fit well between most teeth due to shape. Come in a case that makes it handy to carry around. Give a better tissue massage than interproximal brushes or floss.

Negatives=More likely to splinter and break than round toothpicks. They don't fit into a perio aid.

Go betweens come in a container and are triangular shaped. They are thinner than Stimudents but used the same directional way as them.

Positives=slender and shaped to fit well at gumline between the teeth. Come in a nice case for easy transport.

Negatives=can break or bend with use.

Floss holders come in many sizes and shapes. Some you can replace the floss on, personalizing the type of floss you like to a handle for ease of use.

Negatives=holders that floss is replaced on don't hold the floss tightly so the floss slips off with use. Holds floss straight so can cut your gums if not curved properly.

Positives=easier to floss with a handle.

Listerine or antibacterial mouthwash is the best over the counter mouthwash for killing bacteria. Yes, it is alcohol based and therefore has a slight drying affect but in my experience this is less drying than Peridex which is a prescription mouthwash. It has been shown to help with bleeding gums and plaque/calculus buildup. If overused can cause a yeast infection in the mouth.

Positives=generally kills bacteria that causes bleeding tissues and plaque/calculus.

Negatives=if overused can cause yeast infection in the mouth, also it can be uncomfortable to use if you have xerostomia (dry mouth). Orange or vanilla mint are less "hot" to the mouth.

Toothpicks are the cheapest tissue massagers. They are firm and can be used in a perio aid holder for ease of reaching back teeth.
Positives=cheap, firm, easy to find in stores, easy to carry in wallet, purse, pocket.
Negatives=can be sharp at tip so don't stab yourself. If not on perio aid they are long and can be challenging to reach inside of teeth or even back teeth sometimes.

Plastic picks can be firm tissue massagers. Many times they are rather thin and sharp so be careful. Usually they are handy to carry around so increase chance of use.
Positives=easy to carry around. Provide tissue massage.
Negatives=can be sharp and very thin.

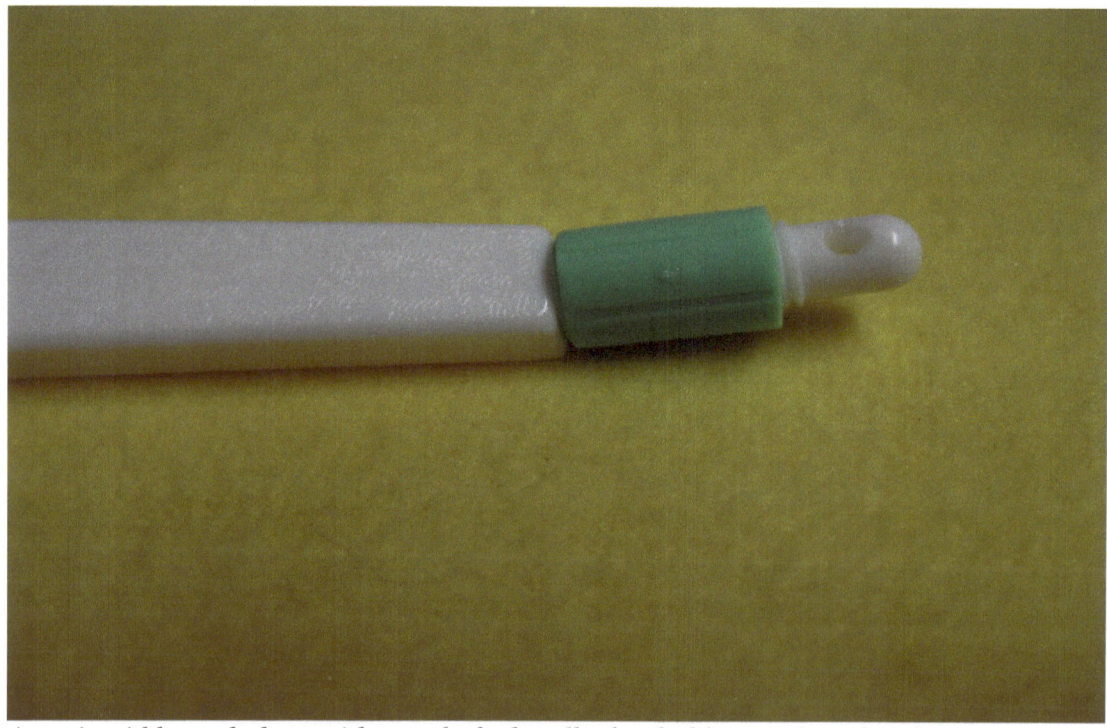

A perio aid has a hole on either end of a handle that holds round toothpicks.

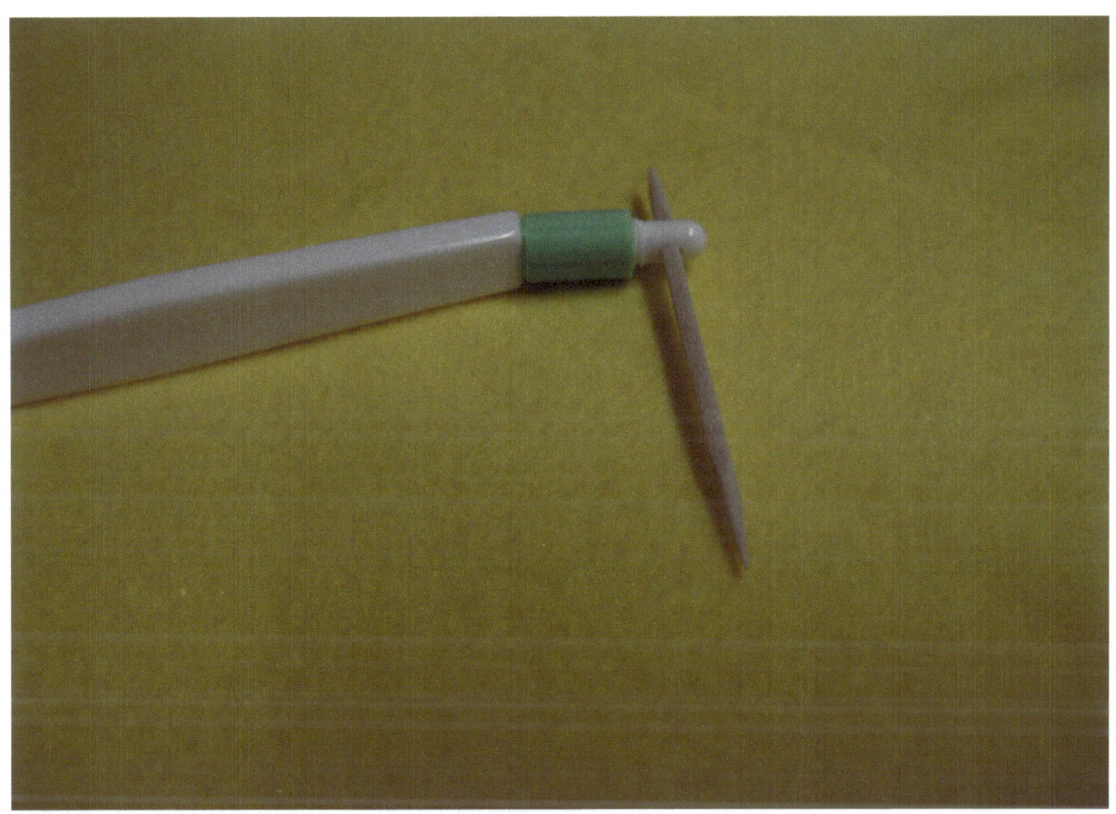

You place a toothpick through the hole and then screw the green portion to apply pressure against the toothpick, holding it in place.

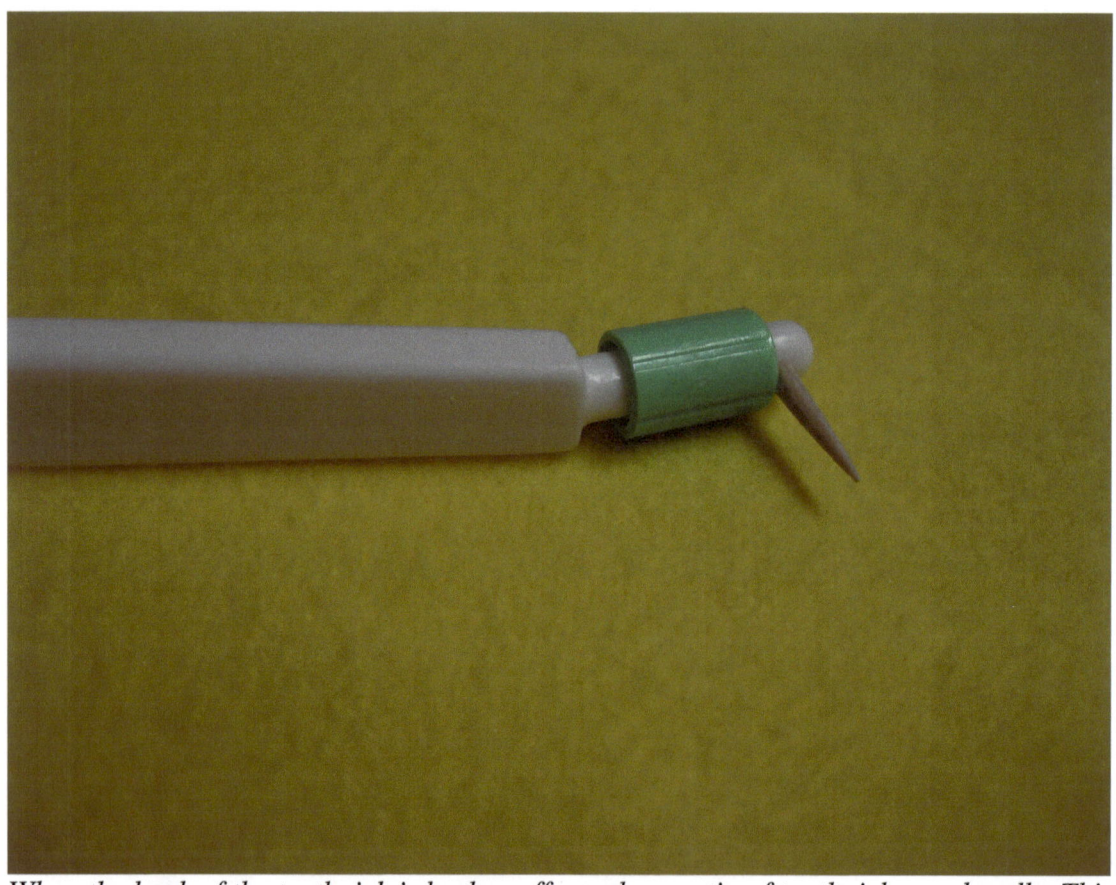

When the back of the toothpick is broken off, you have a tip of toothpick on a handle. This makes it easier to use on the back and inside of teeth.

Perio aids are a handle with holes on either side that hold round toothpicks. You place a toothpick in the end with about 1/3 of toothpick sticking out. You then twist the green pressure tube against toothpick. Then break off the back end of the toothpick leaving a shorter working tool.

Positives=increase ability to reach inside of teeth gum tissues for massage and blood circulation.
Negatives=large tool to carry around. Periodically you have to change the toothpick-sooner if it breaks or splinters.

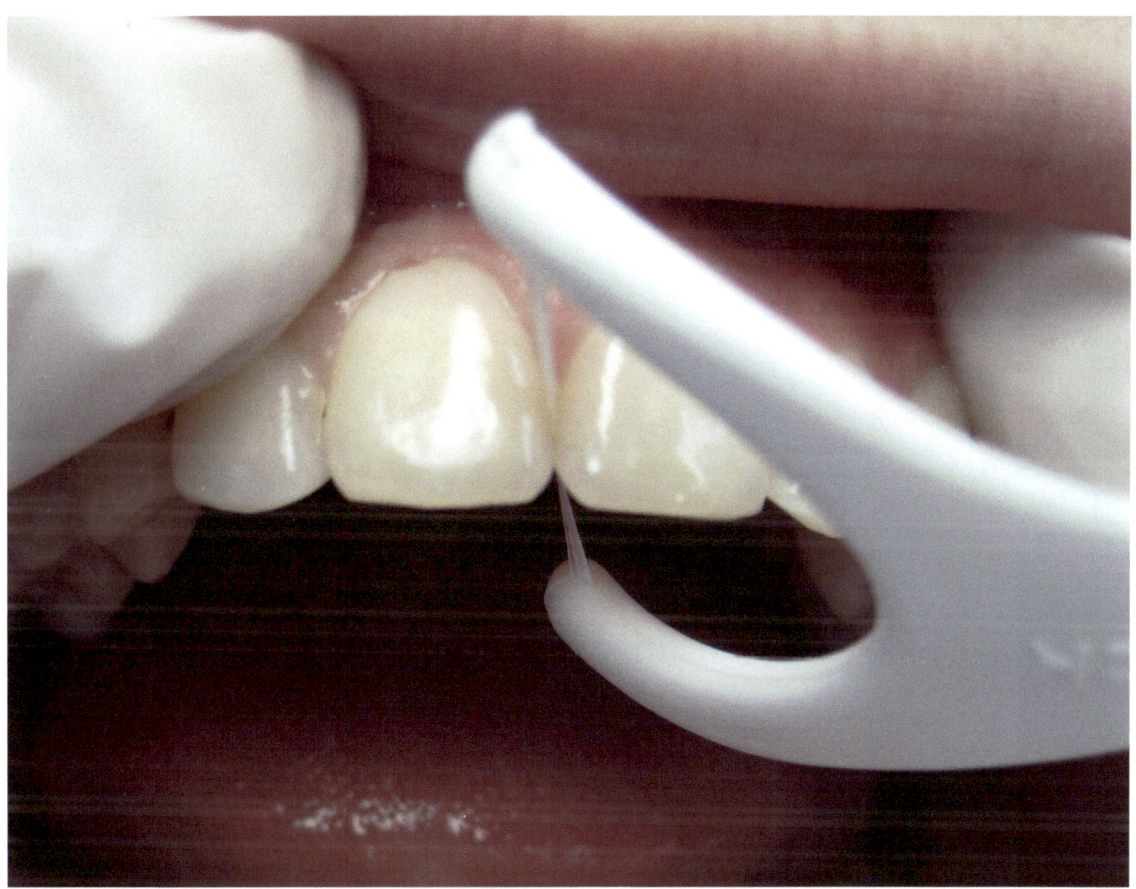

Disposable floss holders come with the floss attached. When using them be careful not to go straight between the teeth. You can see that when the floss is used this way it can cut your gum tissues.

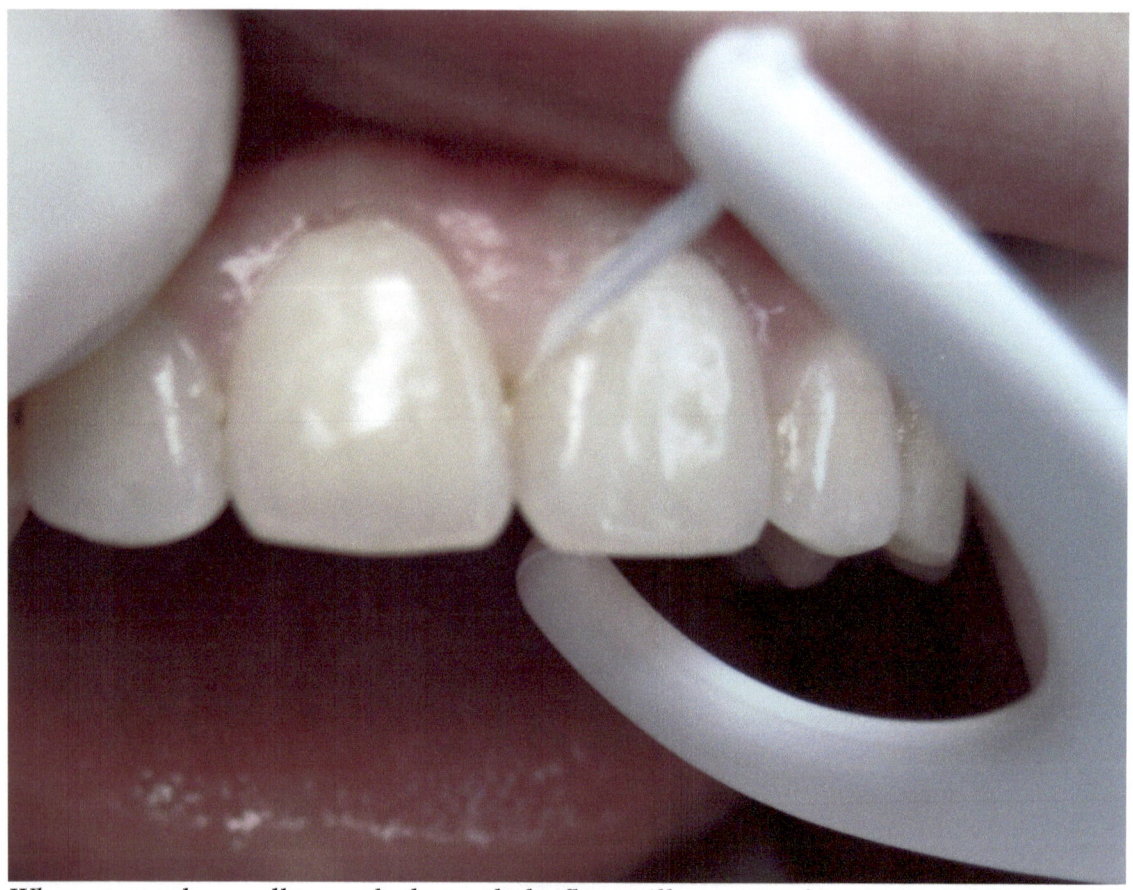

When you push or pull towards the tooth the floss will curve, making it possible to get underneath the gum tissue. That way you can get to the bacteria that cause gum disease and remove them.

Disposable floss holders come in bulk. The handles are plastic and the floss can vary from regular waxed to gortex type. They are reusable and don't have to be thrown away every time you use them. If you rinse them off and let it dry it is fine to use it again because bacteria die with oxygen.
Positives=easier to floss, especially back teeth.

Negatives=holds floss straight so encourages floss cuts in tissue if not curved properly while using. Also people tend not to get under tissues well with this tool so gums don't get massaged as they need, but if you focus on this it can be avoided.

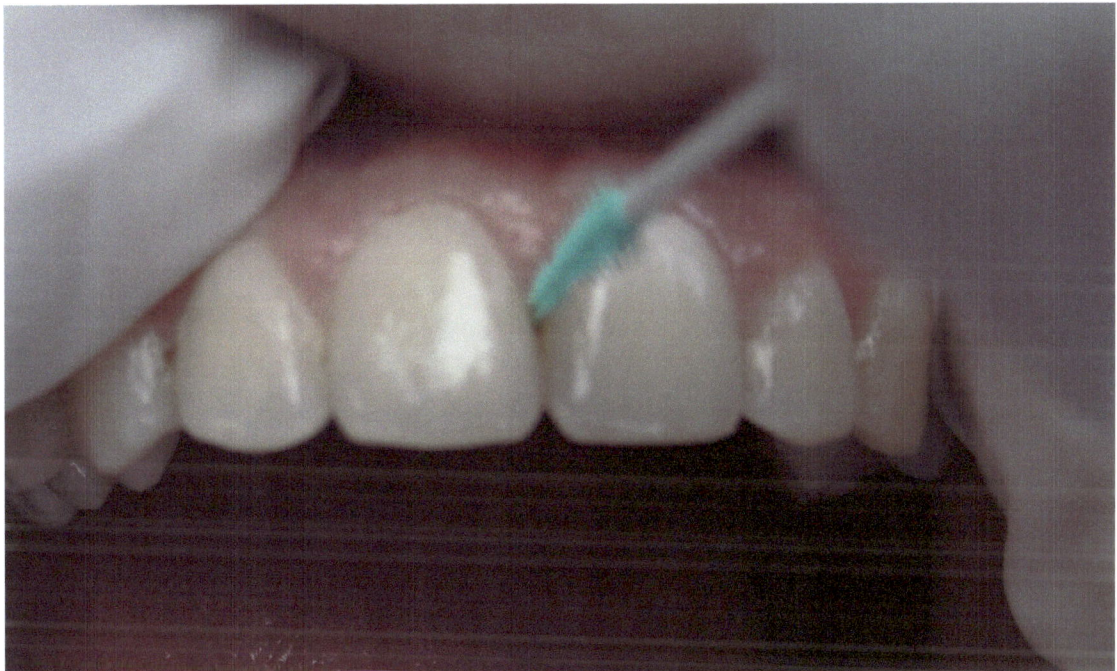

Softpicks are slender and go between the teeth at the top of the interproximal tissue.

Softpicks are relatively new. They are made of rubber and are slender brushes for cleaning between the teeth.
Positives=slender and comfortable to use. Reusable until they bend or break.
Negatives=made of rubber so don't grip teeth as well as sticky tools for plaque removal. Can bend with use.

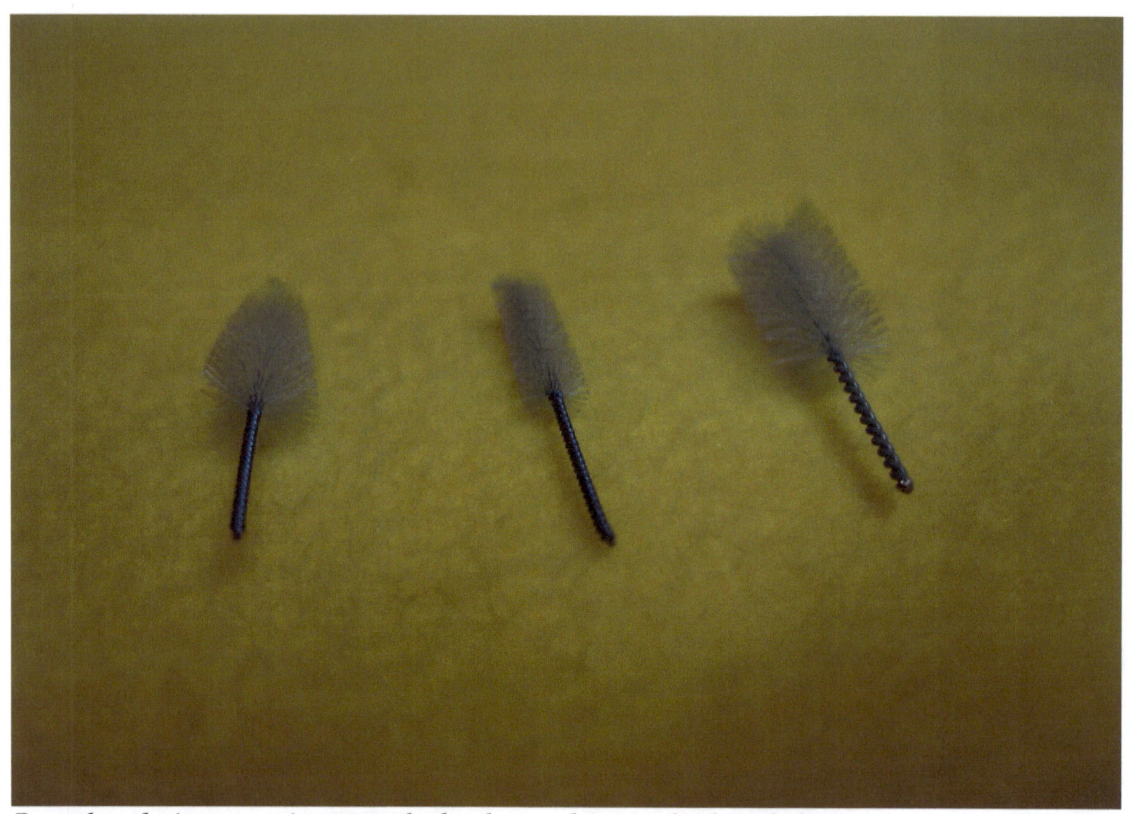

Proxybrush tips some in tapered, slender, or large cylindrical shapes.

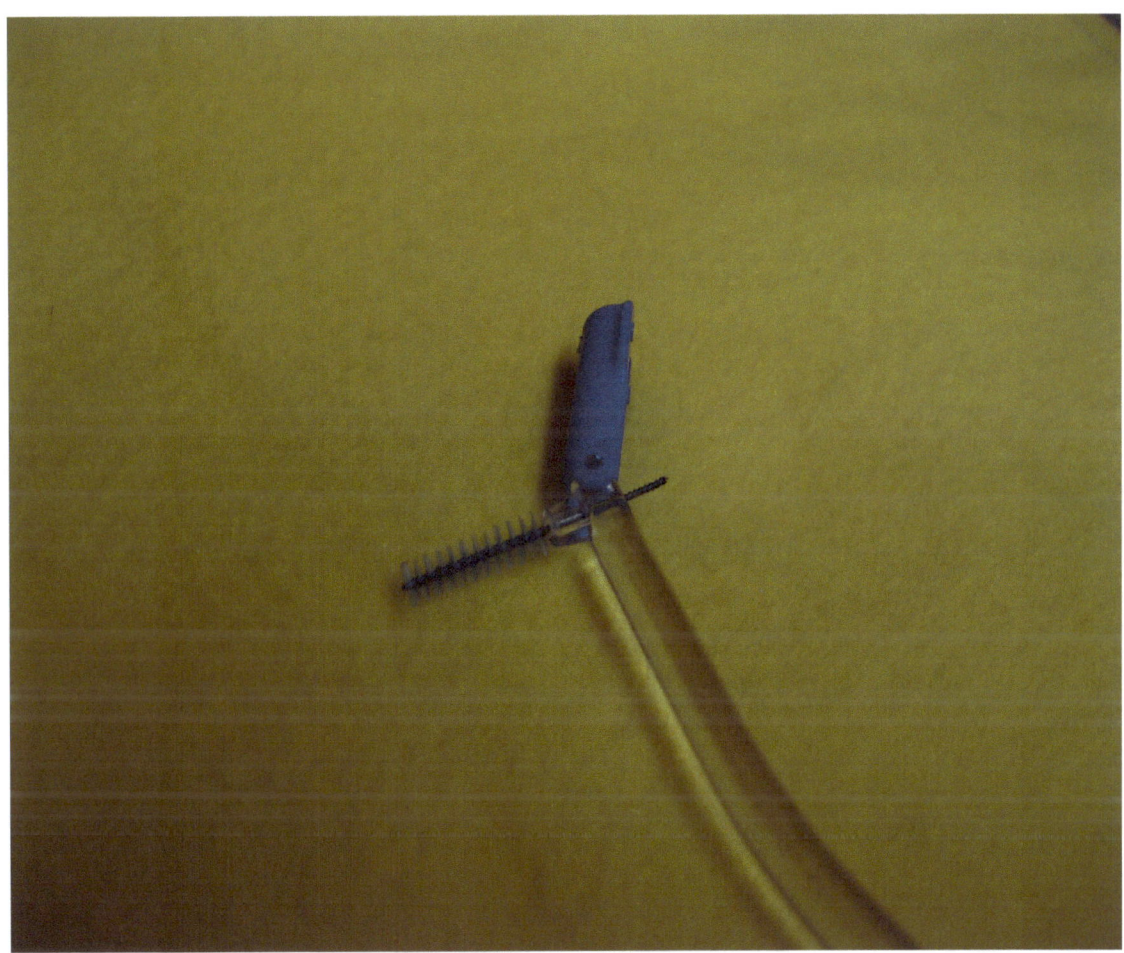

When you place the proxybrush tip into a handle, you then push the blue tip down and it holds the wire brush in place.

Proxybrushes are tools that look like wire brushes, similar to pipe cleaners. They are either attached to a long handle or in a travel sized handle with a lid. They come in slender and large cylindrical shapes, or tapered/Christmas tree shaped.
Positives=brushes between teeth or around bridges/implants.
Negatives=not a firm tissue massage.

Gortex/rubber flosses come in many brand names. Widely used but due to being gortex they are slippery instead of sticky. The ease of getting between the teeth disguises that it also doesn't grip the teeth for good plaque removal. It is good for developing a floss habit in tight contacts, but you should remember what momma always said "if it's easy, it's probably not as worthwhile".
Positives=good for getting between tight teeth, easier to use due to this and encourages the flossing habit.
Negatives=doesn't remove plaque as well as sticky tools do.

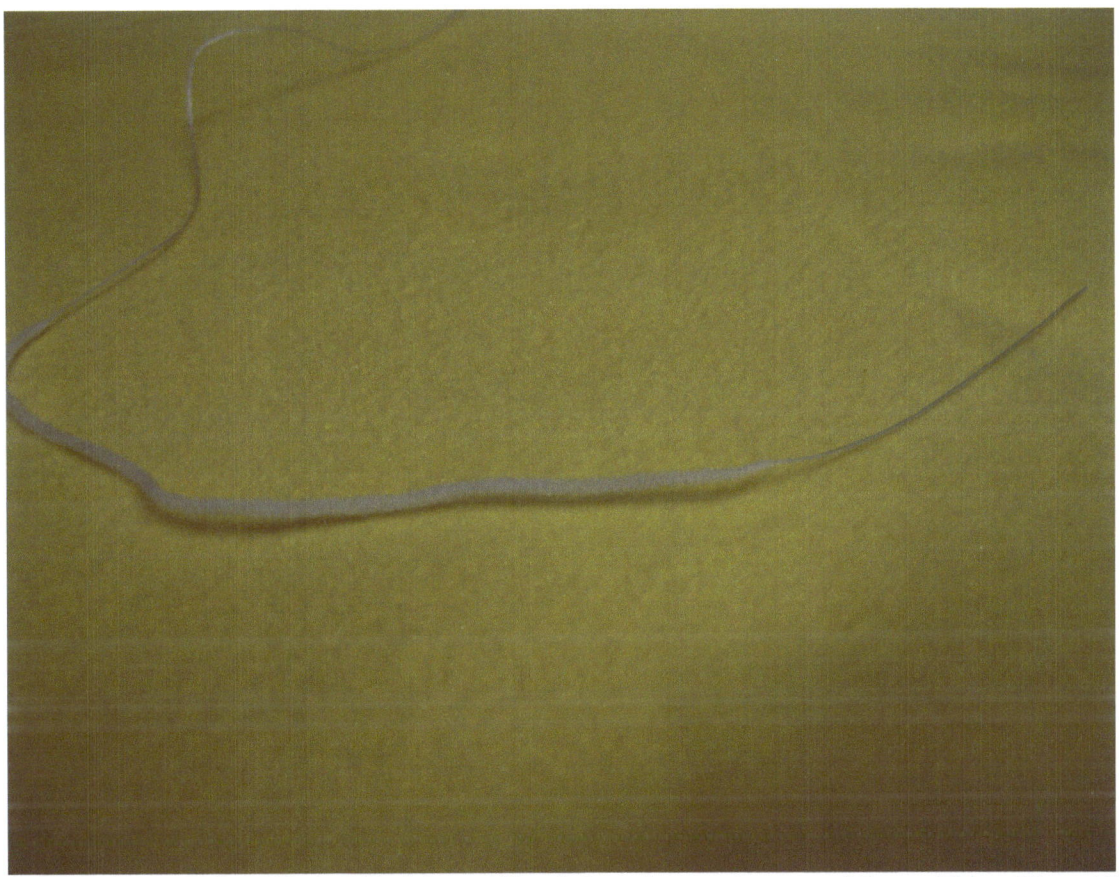

You can see on the right a light blue stiff end then the woven part of Super Floss. The stiff end is to aid in threading under bridges, around fixed retainers, and around orthodontic wires of braces.

Super Floss was created for use under bridges and around braces. It has a light blue stiff end for flossing under areas and a foam/woven area for scrubbing the teeth. This floss is very useful for cleaning in open spaces and behind back teeth as well.

Positives=the foam area has a grittier surface area, even when taut, for removing plaque. Negatives=small working area of foam and rest of floss piece is hard to floss with due to thickness.

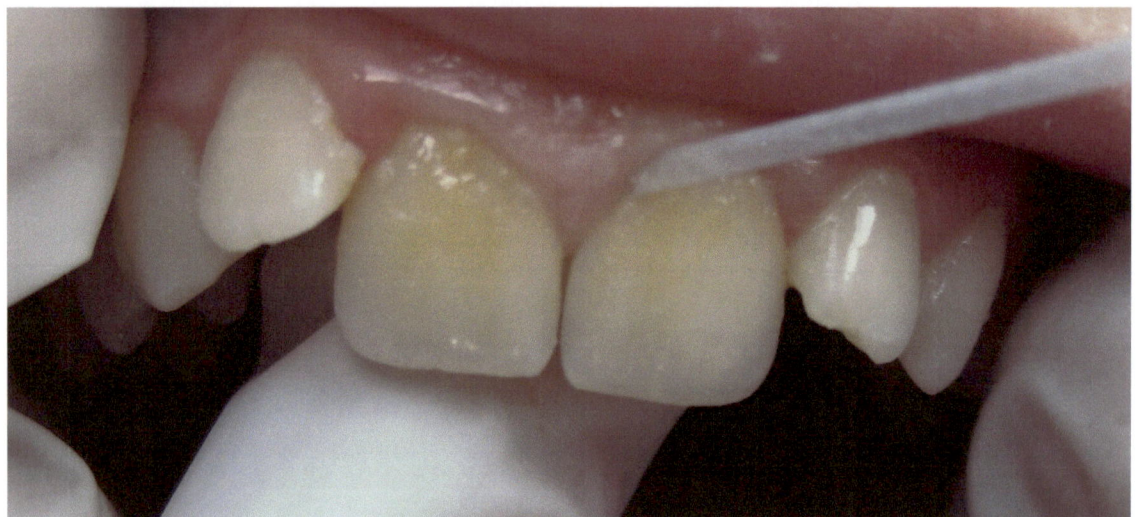

When flossing, remember to take the time to get underneath the gum tissues. When floss is curved well it should be comfortable to do this. If you don't floss underneath the gums then the bacteria living there can still cause gum disease.

Regular waxed floss can be the least expensive way to clean between your teeth with floss. It is sticky and thin. This tool is found everywhere oral hygiene products are sold and doesn't have to be a brand name to be useful.
Positives=easily purchased, works well for average contacts.
Negatives=may be a challenge for tighter contacts.

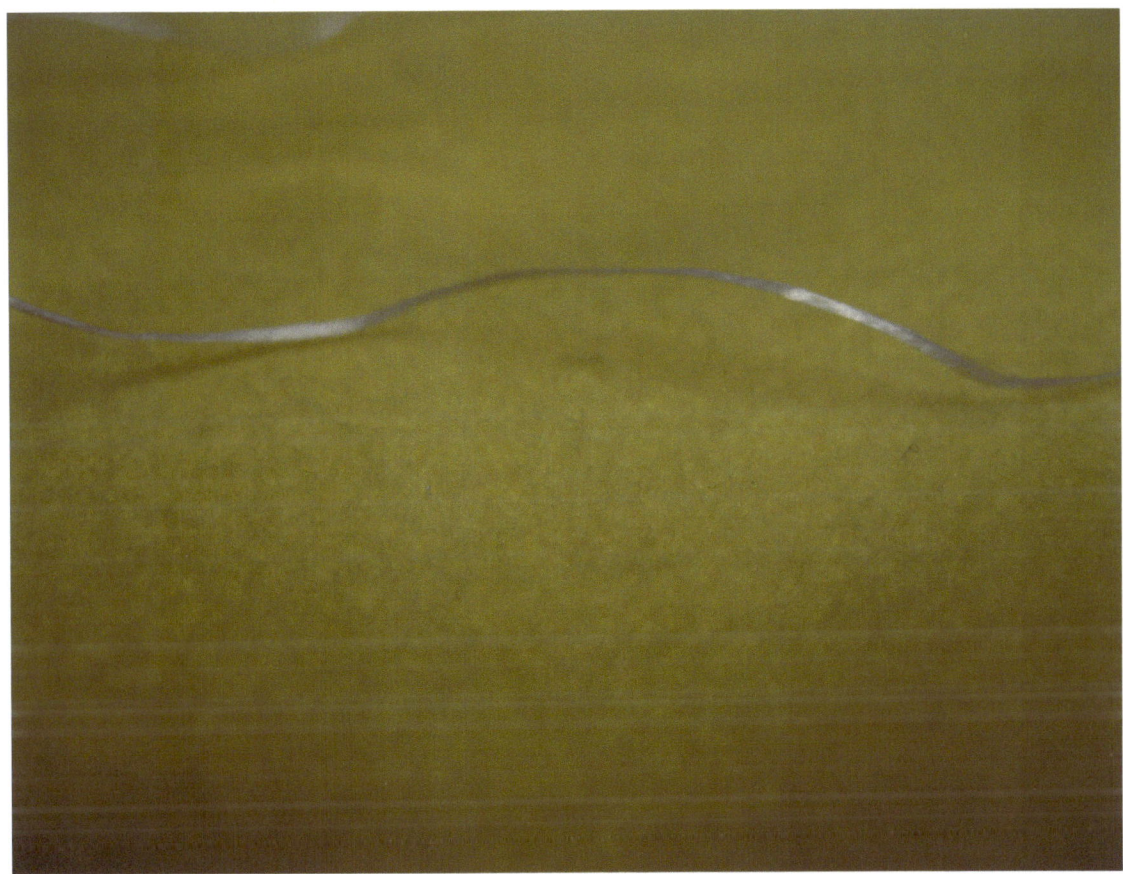

This is a close-up photo of unwaxed dental floss.

Unwaxed floss is ultra thin. Even without wax it grips the teeth for plaque removal.
Positives=tends to work well on tight contacts.
Negatives=due to thin dimensions not as proficient at cleaning open contacts.

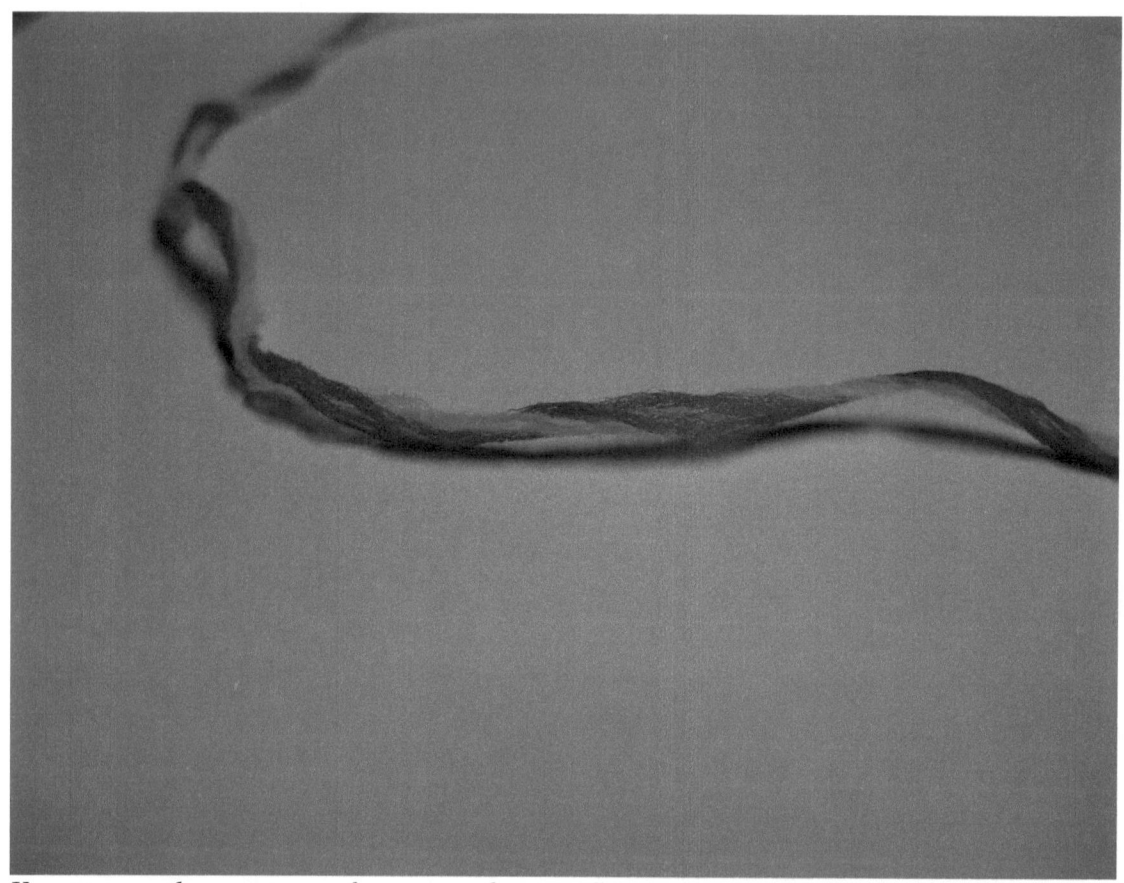

You can see the greater surface area of woven floss compared to the previous photo of unwaxed dental floss.

Woven floss is thicker than regular floss so better for open contacts.
Positives=has more surface area so cleans more tooth surface at once.
Negatives=can shred in tighter contacts leaving "strings" behind.

Dentotape is shaped as it sounds-like ribbon tape. It is heavily waxed and is sticky. This floss is great for open contacts or for getting more tissue massage when flossing.
Positives=better for open contacts and tissue massage.
Negatives=can be too thick for some contacts

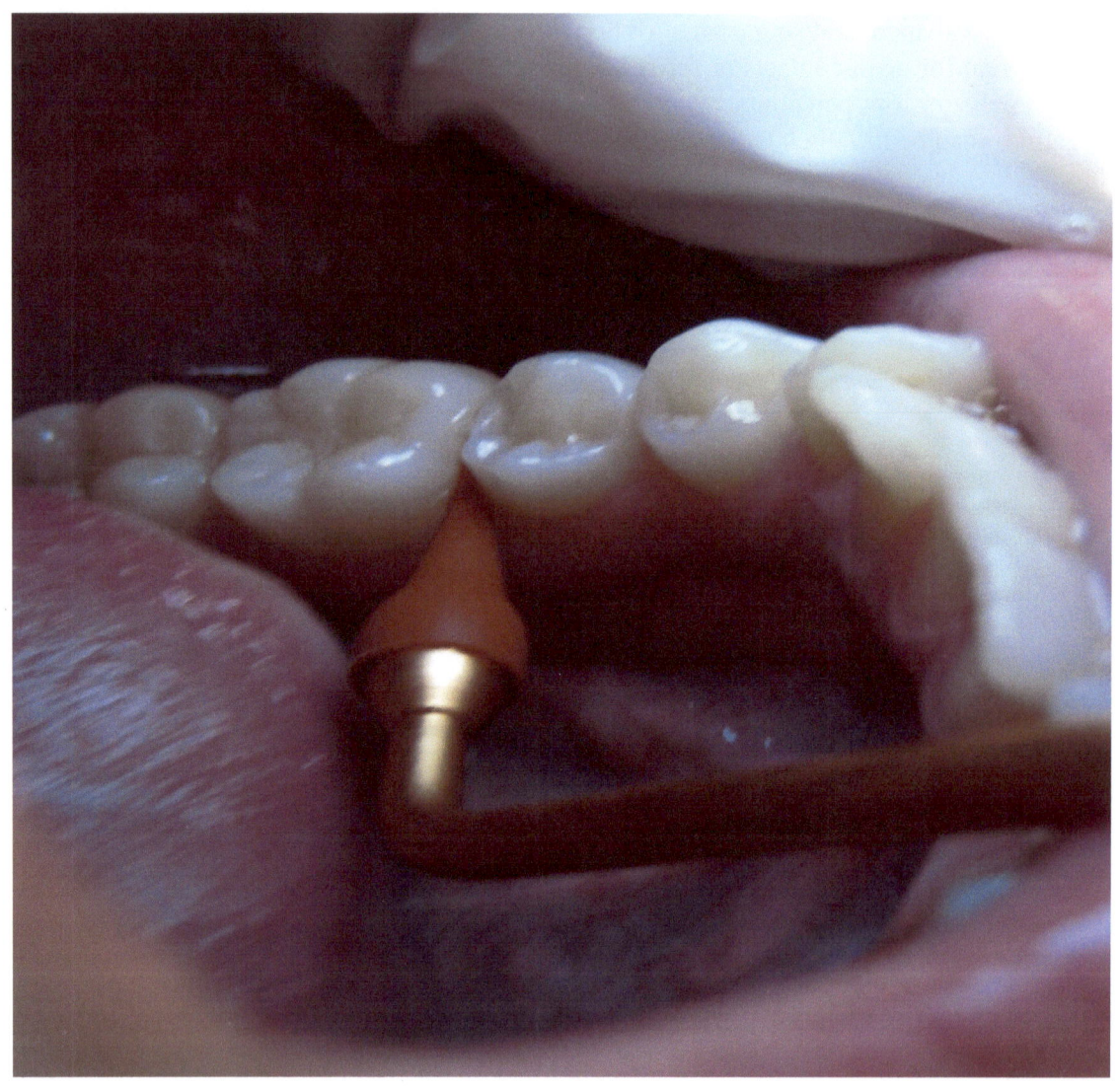

Rubber tip is an oral tool with a handle. The rubber end is great at tissue massage. It can be used for massaging the tissues on the inside of the mouth as well as the outside.

Rubber tip comes on a handle. The rubber tip itself can be replaced when worn out-they become softer with use. Good for tissue massage, although not as firm as toothpicks. Due to handle can be easier to use on inside of teeth gum tissues.
Positives=handle increases chance of tissue massage on inside tissues as well as outside.
Negatives=tips wear out and need to be replaced when they soften. Carrying around the rubber tip is more difficult than some devices for use outside of home.

Peridex or Chlorhexidine gluconate 0.12% is a prescription mouthwash. It has many similarities with Listerine but with a medication that has been shown to kill bacteria that cause periodontal disease. Commonly it is dispensed or prescribed after dental surgeries or in severe gum disease cases.
Positives=strong oral bacteriacidal properties and has been shown to kill periodontal disease causing bacteria.
Negatives=it's a prescription so you need to either get at your dental office or with a prescription. It encourages stain on teeth and changes your taste while using it.

Fluoride rinses/toothpastes over the counter have been shown to be a deterrent of decay if used regularly. Easily purchased at any oral hygiene area of a store goes a long way to help prevent cavities.
Positives=small amount of fluoride that when used regularly helps prevent decay
Negatives=in higher than average caries prone people is not enough to keep cavities from forming.

Prescription fluoride rinses/toothpastes are dispensed or prescribed for highly acidic mouths or people with decay prone oral cavities. Has 10 times the amount of fluoride in them. Fluoride is very water soluble so best to not rinse right after use but expectorate (spit) as much as you want.
Positives=helps to strengthen outside of teeth and can kill bacteria that encourage oral problems.
Negatives=small amounts only are to be used at a time and not rinsing after helps fluoride to stay on teeth longer.

Periostat or Doxycycline 20mg is a form of tetracycline. It is dispensed in a low dose and suppresses the enzyme that causes bone destruction in periodontal disease. It is an anti-inflammatory for the gum tissues. Most recommendations are to take this for a minimum of a year. It is not used to kill bacteria, due to dosage amount; therefore there has been no strengthening of bacteria in the body from this.

Positives=a medication to help with periodontal disease.

Negatives=if not dispensed generic can be expensive. It is like taking a small aspirin for slight blood thinning. Due to it being a form of tetracycline can encourage sensitivity to sunlight. Preferably it is to be taken for a year.

MI paste if rather new. It is made of calcium phosphate which is a natural substance in milk. It coats the teeth and helps to protect teeth from feeling sensations.

Positives=made of natural substance so if swallowed is not harmful. It also comes in multiple flavors.

Negatives=either prescription or dispensed through your dentist.

Sensitivity protection toothpaste comes in many brands-each one using a different chemical for desensitizing the teeth. Used to recommend using for less than a month but no longer have this on the label.

Positives=easy to purchase, over the counter.

Negatives=tend to have less strong flavors to them, but this can be a positive for some people.

Whitening toothpastes have larger pieces of silica as well as some bleaching material in them.

Positives=can lighten teeth some without using bleach treatments.

Negatives=abrasive and can increase sensitivity or wear on teeth.

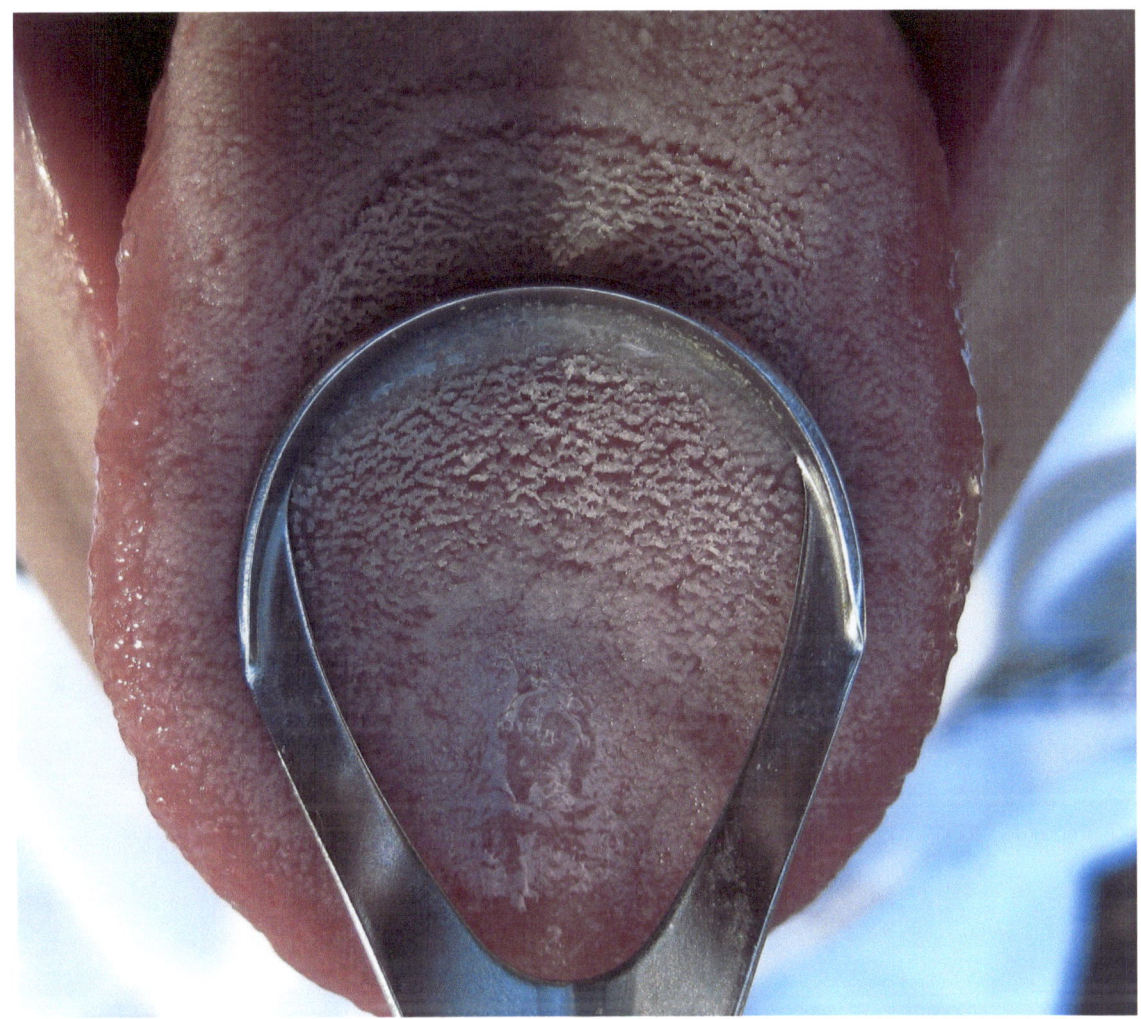

Tongue scrapers come in many shapes and sizes. When used they remove the plaque, food, and bacteria that develops on the top surface. This debris can be a major cause of halitosis or bad breath.

The Humming bird flosser is a slender plastic toothpick at the end of a wide handle that vibrates when turned on. It is easy to use and provides blood circulation to the interproximal tissues.

Positives=easy to use. Wide handle helps people with dexterity problems to clean between their teeth.

Negatives=hard to carry around for use outside the home.

Water picks can remove food debris but not any plaque that's attached to the teeth. It is a good way to irrigate around braces and introduce mouthwash or water under tissues.

Positives=great at removing general debris between the teeth and getting mouthwash underneath tissues.

Negatives=doesn't remove plaque attached to the teeth.

DENTAL CODES AND TREATMENTS

CDT code 4910 Periodontal maintenance is the treatment provided by a dental professional following scaling and root planing. It includes the removal of calculus, plaque, bacteria from above and below the gumline. The frequency of this procedure is to be determined by the professional caring for you. The time between these dental visits varies depending on periodontal pocket depths, amounts of calculus that build between visits, and the patient's oral hygiene care.

CDT code 1110 Adult prophylaxis are the polishing and light scale above the gumline for people aged 14 years old or above provided by dental professionals. On average the entire visit takes about an hour with the cleaning portion varying in time depending on the needs of the patient. Many times this visit will accompany a dental exam. This is an evaluation done of your gum tissues, periodontal bone levels, decay, and general oral and head/neck health. Oral hygiene advice is provided to encourage a healthier oral environment for the individual patient. We aim to educate you about your mouth, including negative issues that are there or developing and try to encourage helpful homecare techniques and tools to help with these.

CDT code 1120 Child prophylaxis are polishing and light scale above the gumline appointments for children, typically aged to 14 years old. They usually take less time than an adult prophylaxis, depending on the need of the patient. These treatment times include generally the same treatment as an adult prophy and accompany a dental exam.

CDT code 4341 for 4 or more teeth, 4342 for 1-3 teeth Scaling/root planning is the treatment provided to a patient with periodontal disease. Generally this is the first treatment done when a patient has deeper pocket depths than the patient can clean well, large amounts of calculus, and/or sensitivity with scaling. Calculus and roughness on the tooth and roots is smoothed with tools. Sometimes localized anesthetic is given, or a topical numbing agent can be used, as well as nitrous oxide for relaxation. Some patients have this treatment without any anesthetic and do fine. The amount of time spent on this procedure is different per patient based on their needs. Commonly 4 hours are needed altogether, 1 hour per quadrant at either 1 or 2 hour intervals for quadrants with 4 or more teeth, sometimes less for 3 or less teeth.

CDT code 4381   Localized chemotherapeutic agents can be placed under gingival tissues for killing bacteria that cause periodontal disease. These vary in form (powder, disc, gel) and type of medication that makes up the product. These are placed with the patient's permission and generally then guided to avoid thoroughly flossing/picking at this area for a week to 10 days so the antibiotic can stay in pocket, killing the oral bacteria there. This can encourage tissues to decrease in swelling, making it easier for the patient to kill bacteria hiding in the periodontal pocket.

CDT code 4210 for 4 or more teeth per quadrant or 4211 for 3 or less teeth   Gingival curettage is the removal of gingival tissues to encourage a healthier mouth. When the periodontal pocket depths are too deep for you to remove bacteria from, an option is to have this extra tissue removed. The gingival tissues can grow back so a change in home care is usually encouraged.

CDT code 1351   Sealants are recommended to cover the grooves on the top of the back teeth with a solid material. This way the bacteria that would live in the deep vaginations of the tooth can be brushed off.

CDT code 4271   Grafting attached tissues is done when the attached tissue, thick, firm, pink instead of red and loose, is not enough to keep the tooth healthy.

CDT code 4260 for 4 or more teeth per quadrant, 4261 for 3 or less   Bone grafts are placed by surgeons where permanent bone loss has occurred to the point of poor prognosis for keeping the tooth long term. Commonly done in single sites where severe bone loss is.

Fluoride treatments have been shown to be an important part of helping to prevent decay. It can be provided to adults (CDT code 1204) children (CDT code 1203), or a fluoride varnish (CDT code 1206) can be applied for desensitizing or because it stays on the teeth longer than a rinse or foam in trays.

CDT code 4355   Full mouth debridement is the removal of calculus that takes longer than the standard amount of time allotted for an adult prophy. Insurance may not cover this procedure so call your insurance if this is recommended.

There are multiple ways to be comfortable for dental treatment. Everyone knows about localized anesthetic, but there are other less invasive options that can give some level of help for discomfort. Nitrous oxide is a gas that is breathed in during treatment. It is commonly called laughing gas, although if you're laughing it's a sign that the nitrous percentage is too high. There is usually a cost for this and most insurance companies don't pay for this (CDT code 9230) but it is the only way some anxious patients will have dental treatment done.

X-rays are the only way we can see cavities between the teeth, bone loss, abscesses, tumors, hidden teeth in the bone, and many other abnormalities that just looking in the mouth we would miss. With the digital x-rays the amount of radiation has decreased quite a bit, not that analog x-rays use a lot of radiation. The full mouth series of xrays (CDT code 0210) are a set of 18 individual films that show, close to the teeth, all roots and in between all teeth. The panelipse x-ray (CDT code 0330) is less radiation than a full mouth series but considered the same by insurance as far as frequency allowed. The panelipse or panorex is a general view of the mouth, sinuses, tempromandibular joint, nasal cavities, and roots of teeth. Typically this view is not clear enough for decay detection. Bitewing x-rays can be 2 (CDT code 0272)=1 on each side, 4 (CDT code 0274)=2 on each side that check for decay between the back teeth, or 7 (CDT code 0277)=2 on each side and 3 for the front teeth.

CDT code 4320   Teeth can be splinted when periodontal disease has progressed to the point of teeth being loose. The dental professional places either a wire or just composite material that holds the teeth in place. By keeping them from moving the teeth are more usable for chewing and stable for longevity.

www.ingramcontent.com/pod-product-compliance
Lightning Source LLC
Chambersburg PA
CBHW041508280526
45792CB00004B/1184